The Healthy
Heart
Miracle

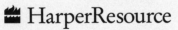 HarperResource

An Imprint of HarperCollins*Publishers*

The Healthy
Heart
Miracle

Your Roadmap
to
Lifelong Health

Gabe Mirkin, M.D., *and* Diana Mirkin

A LINX BOOK

HarperCollins books may be purchased for educational, business, or sales promotional
use. For information please write: Special Markets Department, HarperCollins
Publishers Inc., 10 East 53rd Street, New York, NY 10022.

FIRST EDITION

DESIGNED BY DEBORAH KERNER

Library of Congress Cataloging-in-Publication Data

Mirkin, Gabe.
    The healthy heart miracle : your roadmap to lifelong health / Gabe Mirkin and Diana
Mirkin—1st ed.
        p. cm.
    "A Linx book."
Includes bibliographical references and index.
    ISBN 0-06-019680-7
    1. Heart—Diseases—Prevention. 2. Heart—Diseases—Nutritional aspects. 3. Exercise.
I. Mirkin, Diana. II. Title.

RC682.M575 2004
616.1'205—dc22

                                                                        2003056766

04 05 06 07 08 WBC/RRD 10 9 8 7 6 5 4 3 2 1

To our mother, Vera,

who celebrates her ninety-ninth healthy birthday this year;

to our children, Gene, Jan, Jill, Geoff, Kenny, Peter, Matthew, Amy, and Chris;

and to our grandchildren, Aubrey, Maggie, Kelsey, Thomas, Caroline, Kelly, Paige, Max, Alexandra, Mac, and Owen.

Contents

Before You Begin This Book

I led my medical school class in cholesterol. I was 22 years old, skinny, and otherwise healthy, but my cholesterol level of 300 was worse than that of an out-of-shape 60-year-old. I was headed for a heart attack and that scared me. I began a lifelong quest to lower my cholesterol and to keep it down.

I started taking a new drug, MER-29, but when I read that many people using it developed cataracts, I stopped taking it immediately, and later it was withdrawn from the market. We have much better drugs today, but even the best ones have side effects that can be annoying or keep you from exercising. I knew there had to be a better way.

I enjoyed running, so I started running more than 100 miles a week. I thought I was supposed to run hard every day, so I had one injury after another. And I still couldn't get my total cholesterol under 240.

I started experimenting with my diet. I found that I could keep my LDL, the bad cholesterol, under 100 if I avoided the concentrated sources of calories, saturated fat (in meat, chicken, dairy products, and added fats), and refined grains. I eat all of the whole grains, fruits, vegetables, beans, seeds, and seafood I want.

My running career brought me into contact with experts in exercise science. I began to learn more about training and used my medical knowledge to develop injury prevention and sensible training techniques. My busy medical practice made me focus on devising ways to get the most out of an exercise program. I created and taught a course on sports injuries at the University of Maryland. That led me to write *The Sportsmedicine Book*, which sold almost a million copies. CBS Radio invited me to serve as its fitness commentator, and that led to a daily call-in radio show, which started in 1978. Every weekday for the past 25 years I've talked to callers— as well as to my own patients—about their fitness and health concerns.

The DASH Plus program that I'll explain in this book is the product of all my experiments on my own body and of my study of the large amount of research others have done on diet, exercise, and their effects on heart health. Most important, my program is based on the results I see daily in my patients, and the success stories I hear from listeners and readers who have followed my DASH Plus guidelines.

> ➤ A NOTE FROM DR. GABE
>
> Throughout this book I reference the DASH diet. The DASH study (Dietary Approaches to Stop Hypertension), supported by the National Heart, Lung, and Blood Institute (NHLBI), showed that diet alone can lower blood pressure in 80 percent of people with hypertension. MY DASH Plus program follows the original DASH diet guidelines, with modifications and additions that address total heart health.

THE HEALTHY HEART MIRACLE

The miracle of my DASH Plus program is your body's great capacity to repair damage and revitalize itself even after years of abuse or neglect. Ideally, you would maintain your muscle strength and optimum weight from adolescence onward. But if you have not, it's never too late to make the lifestyle changes that will lower blood pressure, control cholesterol, prevent or reverse diabetes, and make your heart strong enough to have a fighting chance against infections and the stresses of your daily life.

It's better to learn from other people's mistakes than from your own. Some people who have a heart attack or stroke get a second chance, but for others, the warning comes too late. If you're on the road to a heart attack, my 8-Week Plan will help you make a U-turn.

Whether you've picked up this book because of your doctor's warning, the illness or death of a loved one, yet another report in the media about the high rate of heart attacks and strokes, or just as a resolution for a healthier you—any reason is a good reason to commit to a healthy heart lifestyle.

Which of these statements best describes you?

I'm standing on the edge of a cliff. ❑

If you have had a heart attack or stroke, or have diabetes that is out of control, or have had bypass surgery or other procedures to unblock clogged arteries, your life is in jeopardy. I think you also belong in this group if you smoke or are more than 100 pounds overweight. You need immediate, major lifestyle changes. If you want to see your grandchildren grow up and you want to dance at their weddings, give the 8-Week Plan your full attention.

I have one or more warning signs, but no heart-health crises yet. ❑

If you have high blood pressure, high cholesterol, or diabetes; are overweight; store fat primarily in your belly area; or have a family history of heart attacks or diabetes, your doctor has probably warned you of your high risk. In this book you'll learn more about these and other factors, and what you can do about them. You can change the odds—the sooner the better.

I'm basically healthy and want to stay that way.   ☐

Good for you. The 8-Week Plan will help you map out a plan of action that is easy, fun, and tailored to your specific needs. Investing in a healthy heart lifestyle now will pay big dividends in the future.

Wherever you are today, you'll be way ahead at the end of your 8-Week Plan. Each week I'll give you an action program that you can customize to your own situation, needs, and goals. If you are in the "basically healthy" group but have a loved one "with warning signs," or who is "standing on the edge of a cliff," I'll give you lots of ways you can help support him or her and a Personal Roadmap for your loved one (see page 167).

I'm not alone in suggesting that you can make dramatic progress in such a short time:

- A report from the *Journal of the American Medical Association* shows that in just four weeks, a fiber-rich, mostly vegetarian diet can lower blood levels of LDL cholesterol as much as a popular statin drug. The study also showed that the diet lowers C-Reactive Protein levels, a sign of inflammation which is a predictor of heart attacks.
- A study from New Zealand shows that it takes only two weeks for a diet to lower cholesterol as much as it is going to. Many people think that it takes months for a cholesterol-lowering diet to work, but this study confirms what many other studies have shown: Changes in your diet are reflected in your cholesterol numbers within a few days.
- A study from UCLA shows that three weeks of a diet and exercise program can markedly reduce risk factors for heart attacks. In this

study eleven men started a diet and exercised daily for 45 to 60 minutes. Just three weeks later, their systolic and diastolic blood pressures, their total blood cholesterol and LDL cholesterol, and their fasting insulin levels dropped significantly, and they had lost weight.

These and many other studies show that you can improve your heart-health status very quickly with lifestyle changes alone. The improvement continues as you gradually lose excess weight, build endurance, and strengthen your skeletal muscles (and by doing so strengthen your heart muscle). My DASH Plus program is easy to start and simple to follow for the rest of your life. Almost immediately, you will:

- Reduce your chances of suffering from a heart attack, diabetes, stroke, and other diseases
- Lower your blood pressure
- Lower your total LDL (bad) cholesterol level
- Increase your HDL (good) cholesterol level
- Lose excess weight
- Enjoy increased energy, sleep better, and feel great

A QUICK LOOK AT THE PLAN

The 8-Week Plan is based on the DASH Diet, which has been proven to lower blood pressure in 80 percent of people with high blood pressure. My DASH Plus guidelines follow all of the blood-pressure lowering features of the original DASH Diet, while adding other heart-health benefits. Here's what a typical day on the DASH Plus plan looks like:

Whole grains (no limit)
At least 5 servings vegetables
At least 5 servings fruits
Up to 3 servings fat-free dairy products

Up to 2 servings seafood
Beans or legumes (no limit)
1 to 2 tablespoons nuts or seeds
Up to 3 teaspoons olive oil (optional)
Minimal added sugars
MOST IMPORTANT—Exercise! DASH around!

These are guidelines for heart-healthy food choices. Serving sizes of foods in the DASH Plus guidelines are typically ½ cup cooked food or 1 cup raw food, but this is not a portion-control diet; there is no need to measure your food. If you already know that you are at increased health risk, I recommend that you follow these guidelines strictly until your risks are reduced. If you are basically healthy and want to stay that way, you can use the guidelines to fill most of your plate with these good foods and then add whatever else you like.

The 8-Week Plan explains the latest research on how diet and exercise keep your heart healthy and prevent the "diseases of Western civilization" (heart attacks, strokes, diabetes). I'll show you how to shop and how to prepare delicious, easy meals. If you're not exercising now, I'll teach you how to start safely. If you're already involved in a fitness program, I'll show you how to get the most out of your favorite activities. You'll improve your level of fitness whether you're a beginner or an experienced athlete.

The 8-Week Plan is organized in a workbook format so you can enter your results, check your progress, and concentrate on the topics that interest you most. Each week focuses on a different aspect of heart health, and is divided into three parts: Heart-health concepts, Fitness, and Food.

In the first week, I'll explain what tests you need in order to understand your heart health status. The results may be included in reports you've already received from your doctor. If you haven't had any tests taken recently, I'll suggest which ones you should request. You'll also assess your level of fitness as well as lay the groundwork for some changes in your kitchen.

I'll then tell you what your test results mean and get you started on two weeks of my dramatic SHOW ME! Diet. You may be startled by what I ask you to do, but I'm going to PROVE to you, and to your doctor, that you CAN lower your blood pressure, cholesterol, and triglycerides with food. You'll pick your sport and get started on your fitness program, too. At the end of the second week you'll recheck your blood pressure, cholesterol, and triglycerides.

As the weeks go by, you'll get practical tips for controlling blood sugar, cholesterol, and blood pressure. I'll cover the latest theories about inflammation or infection and heart attacks, and how you can apply this information to reduce your risk. All the while I'll be teaching you training principles from competitive athletes and showing you how to make heart-healthy meals that also taste great.

➤ **A NOTE FROM DR. GABE**

Please use a HIGHLIGHTER MARKER to mark up this book! Highlight any of the text that applies to you, and when you fill out the charts, highlight the test results and goals that need your future attention.

The eight weeks will pass quickly, and at the end you'll do another check of any of your tests that had abnormal results. I think you'll be amazed at the change. All of this information can be recorded in your personal plan so that you can refer to it and recheck your progress. Most important, by the end of the eighth week you will have a roadmap—a personal lifestyle plan with all the tools you'll need to stay heart-healthy for life.

Let's get started!

WEEK 1

What's Your Risk?

Ahealthy heart and a strong, lean body go together. If you gain weight over the years or become less fit, you increase your risk for a heart attack, stroke, and other heart-health problems. Heart disease is the number one killer in North America—for both men and women. Your risk soars if you are obese, diabetic, or have high blood pressure or high cholesterol.

Your doctor may already have warned you that you have one or more risk factors for a heart attack or stroke. My 8-Week Plan will show you how to reduce your risk and increase your chances to live a long, healthful life. But first you need to understand your heart-health status and know what questions to ask your doctor. Call and ask your doctor to order the following tests (or ask for copies of the results, if you have had these tests done recently):

HDL and LDL cholesterol (Lipid Panel)
Triglycerides
C-Reactive Protein (CRP)
Lp(a)

Homocysteine
Hemoglobin A1C (HBA1C)
Blood pressure

If your health insurance does not cover some or all of these tests, I think it is worthwhile to cover the cost yourself. Many labs provide the service directly to consumers, but they recommend that you check with your doctor to help you interpret the results.

WHILE YOU'RE TALKING TO YOUR DOCTOR, GET CLEARANCE TO START AN EXERCISE PROGRAM OR TO PICK UP THE PACE OF YOUR CURRENT PROGRAM. When you get your test results, enter them in the Before and After Progress Worksheet on page 250. I'll explain more about what these tests mean in Week 2.

MEASURE YOURSELF

If you are overweight, you probably know it already, and your doctor has probably warned you about the dangers. Before you start my 8-Week Plan, use these three simple measures to see whether you should be concerned about excess weight. You will use this information along with your blood test results to map out a personal heart-health plan.

- Your Body Mass Index (BMI)
- Your Waist/Hip Ratio—to determine whether you're an "apple" or a "pear"
- The "Inch of Pinch" test

Muscle weighs more than fat, and some people have larger, heavier bones than others. You can be heavy and perfectly healthy if a large percentage of your weight is in bone and muscle. However, if a high percentage of your weight is fat, you are at increased risk for diabetes, heart disease, stroke, some types of cancer, and other health problems.

WHAT'S YOUR BMI?

The BMI (Body Mass Index) is a standard calculation used by doctors and nutritionists to determine if your weight is appropriate for your height. To use the chart:

- Locate your height in the left column.
- Follow the row across until you find the weight closest to your weight.
- The number at the top of that column is your BMI.

BMI	19	20	21	22	23	24	25	26	27	28	29	30
Height						Weight (pounds)						
4'10"	91	96	100	105	110	115	119	124	129	134	138	143
4'11"	94	99	104	109	114	119	124	128	133	138	143	148
5'	97	102	107	112	118	123	128	133	138	143	148	153
5'1"	100	106	111	116	122	127	132	137	143	148	153	158
5'2"	104	109	115	120	126	131	136	142	147	153	158	164
5'3"	107	113	118	124	130	135	141	146	152	158	163	169
5'4"	110	116	122	128	134	140	145	151	157	163	169	174
5'5"	114	120	126	132	138	144	150	156	162	168	174	180
5'6"	118	124	130	136	142	148	155	161	167	173	179	186
5'7"	121	127	134	140	146	153	159	166	172	178	185	191
5'8"	125	131	138	144	151	158	164	171	177	184	190	197
5'9"	128	135	142	149	155	162	169	176	182	189	196	203
5'10"	132	139	146	153	160	167	174	181	188	195	202	207
5'11"	136	143	150	157	165	172	179	186	193	200	208	215
6'	140	147	154	162	169	177	184	191	199	206	213	221
6'1"	144	151	159	166	174	182	189	197	204	212	219	227
6'2"	148	155	163	171	179	186	194	202	210	218	225	233
6'3"	152	160	168	176	184	192	200	208	216	224	232	240
6'4"	156	164	172	180	189	197	205	213	221	230	238	246

Source: National Institutes of Health, National Heart, Lung, and Blood Institute

If your BMI is 30 or higher, your risk of death from any cause is increased by 50 to 150 percent. If you are overweight, resolve right now to lose the extra pounds, which will help to reduce your risk of heart attack, stroke, diabetes, and many other health problems. The 8-Week Plan will get you off to a good start.

Record your result on your Before and After Progress Worksheet in the Worksheet section. A healthy weight is an index of 19 to 25, moderately overweight is an index of 26 to 29, and severely overweight is an index higher than 30. Do not use this index if you are pregnant or nursing. If you are a serious athlete, have large muscles, or large bones, see the "Inch of Pinch" test below.

ARE YOU AN "APPLE" OR A "PEAR"?

Some people store fat primarily in the belly area and are called apple shaped, while those who store fat primarily on their hips are called pear shaped. Storing fat primarily in your belly area rather than on your hips increases your chances of suffering heart attacks and diabetes. When you take in more calories than your body needs, your liver turns them into fat. Fat cells stored around your belly are different from those stored on your hips. The blood that flows from belly fat goes directly to your liver, whereas the blood that flows from your hips goes into your general circulation. The livers of people who store fat in their belly area are blocked from removing insulin by the extra fat and therefore do not remove insulin from the bloodstream as effectively as the livers of people who store fat on their hips. So "apples" tend to have higher levels of blood insulin and sugar. You need insulin to drive energy-giving sugar from your bloodstream into your cells. But insulin also lowers blood levels of HDL, the good cholesterol, which prevents heart attacks, and raises blood levels of harmful triglycerides, which cause heart attacks. I'll explain more about the risks of belly fat in Week 3.

Your Waist/Hip Ratio is calculated by dividing your waist size by your hip size. Use a measuring tape to measure your hips at the widest part of your buttocks. Then measure your waist where it is smallest, usually just above the belly button. Then divide your waist measurement by your hip measurement. Record the result on your Before and After Progress Worksheet. Women should have a ratio of 0.8 or lower; men should have a ratio no higher than 1.0. If your ratio is higher than these ideals, you are an "apple" with excess fat stored around your abdomen.

THE "INCH OF PINCH" TEST

Ordinary scales tell you your total weight and can help you keep track of weight changes, but they tell you nothing about the composition of your body. If you are exercising and building muscle, you may gain weight in a healthy way. You can buy special scales that estimate your body-fat percentage, but they are expensive and not completely reliable. Your doctor may use fat calipers or send you for an accurate body-composition test, in which you are immersed in water, but you can make a simple calculation yourself using my "Inch of Pinch" test.

Using your thumb and forefinger, grasp the skin three inches to the right or left of your navel. Pinch firmly but not so hard that it hurts. Then slide your hand away without changing the distance between your thumb and forefinger, and see how far apart your fingers are. Ideally you will have pinched about one-half inch of flesh. An inch or more in your "pinch" means that your excess body weight is more fat than muscle. Record the result on your Before and After Progress Worksheet.

In Week 2, we'll look at what the numbers from your blood tests and blood pressure screening mean. For now, though, whether you are at risk for heart disease, already have heart disease, or are taking a proactive stance (good for you!) in trying to prevent heart disease in yourself and your loved ones, what I recommend will be the same. You will build your own custom heart-health plan to fit your test results and your personal situation, but the basics are the same for everyone: a high-plant diet and plenty of physical activity.

DASH Your Way to Heart Health

I have long advocated a diet made up primarily of fruits, vegetables, whole grains, and beans. Now I'm not alone. Reports published by the Harvard School of Public Health show that a diet rich in plants, with some dairy products, lowers high blood pressure. This is called the DASH (Dietary Approaches to Stop Hypertension) Diet.

Researchers found that it took only two weeks for the DASH Diet to have a dramatic effect on the 459 people taking part in the study. After eight weeks, 70 percent of those following the DASH Diet had normal blood pressure, compared to 45 percent of those who ate only fruits and vegetables, and 23 percent who were given a control diet. The study showed that a diet to lower high blood pressure should be rich in fruits, vegetables, whole grains, beans, seeds, nuts, and low-fat dairy products.

The DASH Diet that was used in these studies is very similar to the lifelong eating habits I'm going to teach you in the 8-Week Plan. I'll explain this further in Week 4. But first, I want you to spend TWO WEEKS on the SHOW ME! Diet, which will prove to you that you CAN lower your blood pressure, cholesterol, and triglycerides with diet alone. This week, while you are getting your tests done, I want you to prepare for two weeks of eating NOTHING but the foods on my Week 2 Menu Plan (page 39). Then—after just two weeks—you will have your doctor re-check your blood pressure and cholesterol, and you'll see the difference. Your doctor will be impressed, too.

First, though, you will need to clean out your kitchen so you'll have no temptation. Plan a shopping trip for the foods you need. You can practice making delicious whole-meal salads using my Mix and Match Salads recipe (page 200). You can also check out your favorite salad bars (in restaurants, delis, or supermarkets) to see how to get a Mix and Match Salad away from home. If you like, go out to dinner the night before you start Week 2. Don't gorge; be reasonable, but eat whatever you like.

KEEP AN 8-WEEK PLAN DIARY

Over the next eight weeks, I want you to keep track of your progress and gather a lot of information you'll want to keep for future reference. Get a notebook or set up a file on your computer to use as a diary. Make a section for your test results and health information, a section for fitness, and a section for food. You can duplicate the forms in the back of the book. You'll also find these and other useful record-keeping tools at www. healthyheartmiracle.com.

DASH Plus Fitness—Week 1: Assess Your Fitness Level

Fitness refers to your heart muscle. The stronger your heart, the more fit you are. The only way to make any muscle stronger is to exercise that muscle against increasing resistance. However, you cannot exercise your heart muscle directly. You can only strengthen this most important muscle in your body by moving your skeletal muscles so your heart works against greater resistance. No drugs strengthen your heart muscle.

Here's the mechanism for strengthening your heart muscle: When you move your legs, your leg muscles squeeze the blood in the nearby veins toward your heart. Then, when your leg muscles relax, the veins fill with blood. This alternating contraction and relaxation of your leg muscles acts as a second heart pushing blood upward. To pump the extra blood from your legs to your heart, and then to the rest of your body, your heart muscle has to contract harder and faster. The harder you exercise, the more blood is pumped by your legs to your heart, and, in turn, the harder your heart has to work to push the blood out to your body. This means that your heart has to beat faster and with more force to do more work.

The strength of your heart and your level of fitness are determined more by how hard you exercise than by how long you exercise, because the harder you exercise, the more blood returns to your heart. This increased amount of blood fills the inside of your heart and stretches it, so your heart has to pump against greater resistance and therefore becomes stronger.

HOW FIT ARE YOU?

Before you can develop your personal DASH Plus Fitness Plan, take this brief quiz to understand your current level of fitness.

A Real-Life Fitness Test*

How old is your body? No, I'm not asking about your age, I'm asking how fit you are for everyday activities. Take this simple test, which covers aerobic capacity, strength, balance, and flexibility. Check the box if your answer is yes.

☐ Can you climb two flights of stairs without getting out of breath?

☐ Do you usually walk down steps without holding on to the railing?

☐ Can you rise from a low chair without using your hands?

☐ Can you put on and tie a shoe while balancing on the other foot?

☐ Can you lift a full carry-on suitcase into an overhead luggage compartment?

❑ Can you do heavy household jobs without feeling sore the next day?

❑ Can you get down on the floor and get up without strain?

❑ When you walk with a healthy friend your own age, do you keep up?

❑ Can you reach all the parts of your body that you need to reach for dressing, grooming, and personal hygiene?

❑ Do you have the energy to enjoy life, to dance at a wedding or play volleyball at a picnic—rather than just being a spectator?

Now count the checks and enter them here _____. That's your score. Here's what it means:

10 You're moving like a person 20 to 39. If you're older than that, congratulations! Stay fit and you can remain youthful for many years.

7–9 Consider yourself middle-aged, fitness wise. You're functioning like someone age 40 to 59. That's great if you're actually a senior citizen. Otherwise, you could do better if you become more fit.

4–6 Your body behaves like the body of a person 60 to 79. This is good if you're over 80. If not, you could turn back the clock by a decade or more if you shape up.

0–3 Your physical limitations are like those of a person age 80 or older. Even people who really are 80-plus can improve their capacity to perform everyday tasks by becoming more fit.

After you've been exercising for a few months, take this test again. You'll be surprised and pleased to see how much difference a regular exercise program can make.

From QUICK FIT by Richard Bradley and Sarah Wernick. Copyright © 2004 by Richard R. Bradley and Sarah Wernick. Reprinted with permission of Atria Books, an imprint of Simon & Schuster Adult Publishing Group.

GETTING STARTED WITH FITNESS

If you already exercise regularly, skip to the Fitness section of Week 3 to learn how to get the most heart-health benefit from your program. Check with your doctor or health care provider before beginning a new exercise program or increasing the intensity of your existing program. Next week you'll get started on a lifetime of fitness and heart health. While you are waiting for your doctor's approval, just try to move around more than you normally do.

MORE TODAY THAN YESTERDAY

The goal for this first week is simply to move more today than you did yesterday, and more tomorrow than you did today. Don't worry . . . this won't be hard, and you may even find that some of the ideas below are fun:

• Park a block from your destination and walk.
• Take the stairs instead of the elevator or escalator.
• Try out some exercise equipment at a store, gym, or exercise room.
• Squeeze a tennis ball.
• Tap your feet in time to music while you work.
• Hang clothes outside to dry.
• Plant some flowers.

- Play an active game with your children, your grandchildren, or someone else's children.
- Drum your fingers or swing your leg while sitting (where you won't annoy anyone).
- Walk around your house (inside or out).
- Vacuum and wash your car.
- Brush your dog.
- Sweep your porch or tackle a cleaning project you've been putting off.
- Go fishing or go to a park with a friend.

Add more ideas of your own. Use the Fitness section of your notebook to jot down your accomplishments. DO NOT try to exercise vigorously for half an hour, twenty minutes, or even ten minutes. If you are out of shape, it's very important to start your new exercise program gradually, and only with your doctor's approval. We'll get started next week.

> **A NOTE FROM DR. GABE**

Get your doctor's permission before starting an exercise program or a strenuous new activity. Many doctors will recommend a stress test.

DASH Plus Food—Week 1: Groundwork

Check with your physician first. If your doctor or health care provider has given you specific diet instructions, or if you have any special dietary requirements, do not make changes to your current diet without his or her approval.

Assess your current eating habits. Write down everything you ate yesterday. Then keep track of what you eat today and tomorrow. Record the foods, amounts, and times you eat. Then compare your diet with the DASH Plus Diet guidelines on page 5. This will help you understand how much, or how little, you may need to change. Did you eat five fruits and five vegetables? Did you eat any whole grains? What foods did you eat that aren't listed?

Now give some thought to your eating patterns: Do you eat when you're hungry or at a specific time? Which foods do you truly enjoy, and which ones do you eat out of habit? Do you eat when you are bored, nervous, or tired? Do you eat in front of the television set or at your desk? The 8-Week Plan doesn't dictate when or why you eat, but if you find it hard to make the changes I suggest, you may want to ask yourself some of the above questions.

CLEAN OUT YOUR KITCHEN

Before you start your two-week SHOW ME! Diet, get rid of any foods that are not on the Food Lists on pages 177–183. This will be hard if you hate to throw things away, but you'll be doing yourself a big favor. It's much easier to avoid temptation if these foods aren't in your kitchen. Take a trash bag or cardboard box and go through your refrigerator, cupboards, and pantry. Get rid of:

Bread, cookies, chips, crackers, and any other bakery products
Pasta, white rice
Flour, corn meal, cake mixes
Any cereals made with refined grains (see healthy choices on
   page 179)
Butter, margarine, lard, Crisco
Any foods containing partially hydrogenated oils (check the list of
   ingredients)
Meat (including chicken and turkey)
Eggs

Ice cream, whole milk, any dairy products except skim milk or fat-
free yogurt

Cheese (you can keep hard grating cheeses such as Parmesan or
Romano)

Salad dressings and mayonnaise (except low-calorie versions)

Any prepared foods or frozen foods that contain the foods listed
above or that have fewer than 3 grams of fiber per serving

Throw all of these out or give them away!

If you have family members who will not be following the SHOW
ME! Diet with you, work out a strategy to keep your temptations to a
minimum. Keep flavors that they like and you hate. Reserve a section of
the refrigerator and a cupboard for yourself and try not to look anywhere
else. Better yet, tell your family to hide their junk food so you won't even
know where it is. I hope the other adults in your household will participate with you. The SHOW ME! Diet will not hurt anyone, and chances
are your spouse will benefit from it, too.

WEEK 1 MEALS

After you write down what you ate for three days, use the rest of Week 1
for shopping and practice. Eat whatever you like, but keep the DASH
Plus Diet guidelines in mind and try to include more vegetables and fruit
in your menus. Try out a few of the recipes at the back of the book if you
like. You'll be ahead of the game if you practice making Mix and Match
Salads, the mainstay of the SHOW ME! Diet you will start in Week 2.
Shop for ingredients using the list below. Then experiment with different
seasonings, vinegars, and low-calorie dressings to find those that taste
good to you.

Now that you've emptied out your refrigerator and cupboards, take a
shopping trip for the foods you will need for Week 2 and later. Don't buy
more fresh produce than you will use in a few days, but you can stock up
on the foods that store well.

> ➤ A NOTE FROM DR. GABE
>
> The DASH Plus Mix and Match Salad is a one-dish meal with endless variations (see page 200). Stock your refrigerator so you can make this fast food often.

SHOW ME! DIET SHOPPING CHECKLIST

For breakfast:

Long-cooking oatmeal: rolled, steel cut, Irish or Scottish style
Raisins or other dried fruits (optional)
Skim milk, fat-free yogurt, or the milk substitute of your choice
Fresh fruits (optional)

For your Mix and Match Salads, pick from these choices or others from the recipe on page 200:

Salad greens such as romaine lettuce
Your choice of other salad vegetables: Whatever appeals to you and looks fresh in your produce department, including tomatoes, avocados, artichoke hearts (sold in jars), red bell peppers
Canned salmon (red sockeye tastes best), canned tuna
Canned beans, canned chickpeas
Nuts, peanuts, soy nuts, sunflower seeds, and other seeds
Grated or shredded hard cheese such as Parmesan or Romano
Mild vinegar such as rice wine vinegar and/or low-calorie dressings
Herbs, spices, and spice blends, such as Cajun spice blend, salad spice mix, or your personal favorites

Miscellaneous:

Calorie-free beverages of your choice, such as water—plain, sparkling, or flavored (tap water is fine, too); tea, coffee, calorie-free iced tea

For a Stock-Up Shopping List that you can take with you to the grocery store, see page 184.

SUPPORT YOUR LOVED ONE

What if the person in your household who needs help the most isn't the least bit interested in eating better? You need a strategy. (That means, be sneaky!) See if you can get your loved one to follow the SHOW ME! Challenge with you in Week 2; that can at least get some discussion going. It helps if you're the one who plans and prepares the meals, but if you're not, take on more of this responsibility. You can announce your plans or just gradually take over and make changes. Do the kitchen cleanout (see page 19) over several weeks, replacing the items that disappear with some interesting new choices from the DASH Plus guidelines. Look through the recipe section and see if you can find some that include ingredients your loved one likes, then add a few new dishes each week. Pack lunches so you can have at least some influence over meals eaten outside the house, but if you can only control most of the breakfast and dinner choices, you'll be making big strides.

It's much harder to make changes in someone else than it is to motivate yourself, but if you're persistent, small changes over time can add up to a big difference in your loved one's health.

CONGRATULATIONS!

You've finished Week 1 of the 8-Week Plan. For many people, that's the toughest hurdle—just getting started. Now that you've made it through the first week it should become even easier as the weeks pass. You're on your way to a healthier heart!

What Do You Test Results Mean?

By now you have the results of the tests you took in Week 1 and have recorded them on your Before and After Progress Worksheet in the Worksheet section. If your doctor is concerned about any of the test results, please explain that you are going to follow a very strict DASH-type diet plan for the next two weeks and ask to be retested then before he or she makes any recommendations about medication or other actions.

Ask for a copy of your lab test reports and keep them in a file for future reference. Labs may use different scales for some tests, but the report will always show the lab's normal range for each test and will flag any of your results that are abnormally high or low. (Canadian values are often different from those used in the United States.)

In the next few pages I'll explain what these tests measure and what your results mean. If any of your numbers are high or abnormal, you may want to read about those tests first, but please don't skip the other test explanations. Your normal results are important for your personal DASH Plus plan, too.

LDL AND HDL CHOLESTEROL

Fat is carried in your bloodstream in little balls coated with protein, called lipoproteins. Your cholesterol test measures the different lipoproteins to help predict your risk for a heart attack. You may have heard that your total cholesterol should not be higher than 200, but doctors now evaluate a ratio between your HDL cholesterol and your LDL cholesterol. Here are some simple guidelines to help you interpret your own numbers.

HDL, the "good" cholesterol, carries cholesterol molecules from your bloodstream to your liver, where they can be removed from your body. LDL, the "bad" cholesterol, carries cholesterol molecules to your arteries, where they may form plaque. To remind yourself that HDL cholesterol is good, remember that H stands for Healthy. To remind yourself that LDL cholesterol is bad, remember that L stands for Lousy.

HDL cholesterol protects you from the LDL cholesterol. If your LDL is 100, you need at least 40 HDL to protect you. If your LDL is 140, you need at least 60 HDL to protect you. Most doctors recommend that an LDL over 140 should be lowered, no matter how high your HDL. You can predict your risk by seeing how your values compare to these:

If your LDL is:	You need an HDL of at least:
90	35
100	40
110	45
120	50
130	55
140*	60

*Most doctors recommend lowering an LDL over 140, no matter how high your HDL may be.

IF YOUR LDL IS TOO HIGH

People with high LDL cholesterol are sensitive to taking in too much fat and too many calories. If your LDL is too high, you need to restrict saturated fats, which are found in meat, chicken, and whole-milk dairy products, and partially hydrogenated fats, which are found in many prepared foods such as French fries, cookies, crackers, and many bakery products. You must also reduce your total intake of calories, which means you should not resort to "low-fat" foods that still contain lots of calories.

IF YOUR HDL IS TOO LOW

People with low blood levels of HDL, the good cholesterol, are sensitive to eating too many calories and too many refined carbohydrates. They are the ones most likely to become diabetic, store fat around their bellies, have little hip fat, and have high blood levels of triglycerides. People with low blood levels of HDL cholesterol should be treated as if they are diabetic. If your HDL is low, avoid refined carbohydrates (foods made with flour, white rice, milled corn, or added sugars) and cut back on your total calorie intake. You can reduce chances of suffering a heart attack by 2 percent for every one-point rise in HDL. If your HDL is low and your triglycerides are high, pay particular attention to the section below on triglycerides.

> A NOTE FROM DR. GABE

Please note: This book is not an encyclopedia of heart problems. If you have been diagnosed with a specific defect or disease and need more information, please check with your doctor. Many Web sites provide additional detailed information (see www.healthyheartmiracle.com).

Tips for Raising Your HDL

- Avoid all refined carbohydrates (flour, white rice, milled corn, all added sugars).
- Lose weight and burn extra calories with exercise. For every pound of fat you lose, you can expect to see a 1 percent rise in your HDL.
- Exercise BEFORE you eat. A study at the University of Missouri shows that exercising regularly before eating raises HDL cholesterol, because exercise stimulates the fat-clearing enzyme lipoprotein lipase, which lowers triglycerides. HDL is used up in clearing triglycerides, so lowering triglycerides raises HDL cholesterol.
- Don't smoke. A study at Vanderbilt University showed that within just one week of quitting smoking, people's HDL levels increased by seven points.

The SHOW ME! Diet that you will start this week works for both high LDL and low HDL. It takes only two weeks to get the maximum cholesterol-changing benefit from any diet. Ask your doctor to recheck your cholesterol after you have followed the SHOW ME! Diet for two weeks with no cheating! I think you will both be delighted with the results. If you are already taking cholesterol-lowering medications, continue them while you follow the SHOW ME! Diet. Your numbers will improve and may help you convince your doctor to try reducing your drugs, or even giving you a trial period without them, using only the 8-Week Plan lifestyle changes. However, if your numbers are still abnormal, you may need to take medication in addition to following a heart-healthy diet. (More on cholesterol in Week 5.)

TRIGLYCERIDES

When you take in more calories than your body needs, your liver converts the extra calories into fat molecules called triglycerides. It doesn't matter whether the extra calories come from carbohydrates, fats, or proteins. After you eat, your blood-sugar levels rise, which causes your pancreas to release insulin that helps the liver convert sugar to triglycerides. If your blood-sugar levels rise higher than normal, you produce large amounts of insulin, which causes your liver to make even more triglycerides. Insulin also lowers blood levels of the HDL cholesterol that helps prevent heart attacks. People with high blood levels of triglycerides often store most of their fat around their bellies rather than on their hips and have low blood levels of HDL cholesterol.

If your triglyceride level is above the norm of 150, it means that you eat too much food or have high blood-insulin levels, which can cause heart attacks. Having moderately elevated blood levels of triglycerides does not increase your risk for a heart attack unless you also have low blood levels of HDL cholesterol. To keep blood-triglyceride levels from rising too high, HDL cholesterol carries triglycerides back to the liver to remove them from the bloodstream. So triglycerides usually do not increase your chances of developing a heart attack until you produce so much that they lower blood levels of HDL cholesterol and clog up your arteries.

You can usually reduce blood-triglyceride levels just by eating less food and avoiding foods that cause the highest rise in blood sugar, such as bakery products, pasta, and foods with added sugar. (More on triglycerides in Week 3.)

BLOOD PRESSURE

Your heart pumps blood through your arteries. The force this creates on your artery walls is called blood pressure. Blood pressure is measured in millimeters when a cuff is tightened around your arm and again when it is loosened. This gives you two blood pressure numbers: systolic, which measures blood pressure when your heart contracts, and the much lower diastolic, which measures blood pressure when your heart relaxes.

When your heart contracts, it pushes a huge amount of blood out to your arteries. Your arteries are supposed to act like balloons and expand to accept the blood and prevent your blood pressure from rising too high. Having plaque in your arteries stiffens them and prevents them from expanding when your heart contracts, causing your blood pressure to rise higher than normal. The stiffer your arteries become, the higher your blood pressure rises. The intense pressure on artery walls from high blood pressure can cause damage that provides ideal places for even more plaque to accumulate. It's a vicious circle—high blood pressure continues to cause plaque buildup, which narrows the arteries and increases blood pressure even more.

High blood pressure, also called hypertension, is one of the primary risk factors for heart disease, yet it can go unnoticed for years because you usually don't feel anything when your pressure is up. The systolic (contraction) blood pressure is more of a concern than the diastolic (relaxation) blood pressure as an indicator of your risk of a heart attack or stroke. Your risk is increased further if you also have high blood cholesterol, sugar, or insulin levels; an enlarged heart; or are overweight. Over time, high blood pressure can cause serious damage to your cardiovascular system, kidneys, and other organs.

If your blood pressure is over 120/80, start the SHOW ME! Diet immediately and then recheck your blood pressure in two weeks. (More on prevention and treatment of high blood pressure in Week 4.)

How High Is Too High?

- 120/80 is normal; lower is better
- Up to 139/89 is considered pre-hypertension ("borderline" or "high normal")
- 140/90 is high (hypertension)

HEMOGLOBIN A1C (HBA1C)

Diabetes that is not tightly controlled puts you at high risk for a heart attack. HBA1C is the most dependable test available to find out if you are at risk for the side effects of diabetes. It is used both to diagnose diabetes and to monitor the progress of a person who has diabetes. Many people do not know they have diabetes and are not diagnosed until after they have a heart attack.

In addition to heart attacks, uncontrolled diabetics are at high risk for strokes, blindness, deafness, burning foot syndrome, impotence, kidney failure, amputations, and damage to any organ or tissue in their bodies. Almost all of these effects are caused by blood sugar constantly rising too high after meals. After you eat, your blood sugar is supposed to rise from a normal level of around 100 to perhaps 160. If it rises higher than that, sugar sticks to cells. Once sugar is stuck on cells it cannot get off; it is converted to a poison called sorbitol that destroys the cells. This destruction causes the horrible side effects of diabetes.

Your blood sugar goes up and down all day long. A single glucose test tells you only what your blood sugar level is at that moment, but HBA1C gives you an "average" reading and tells you how much sugar is stuck on the surface of cells. If your HBA1C level is above the normal 6.1, you are at increased risk for a heart attack and the other side effects of diabetes, even if you have not yet been diagnosed with the disease. If you are a diabetic and your HBA1C is above 6.1, your doctor should evaluate and perhaps change your medication, and you need to be much more strict with your diet. (More on diabetes, insulin, and blood sugar in Week 3.)

CRP (C-REACTIVE PROTEIN)

Recent research shows that having a high C-Reactive Protein blood level increases your risk of suffering a heart attack or stroke by twice as much as having a high cholesterol level. C-Reactive Protein (CRP) measures

The Lowdown on Carbs

Anyone with diabetes, high cholesterol, or high blood pressure should avoid refined carbohydrates. Nature always packages carbohydrates with fiber, vitamins, minerals, and other nutrients. Many of these nutrients are removed when food manufacturers mill whole grains to make flour, or extract sugars from sugar cane and other plants. Foods made with these *refined carbohydrates,* such as bread, pasta, bagels, cookies, and crackers cause almost the same rise in your blood sugar as plain table sugar.

On the 8-Week Plan you will learn to avoid these foods and *increase* your consumption of *unrefined* carbohydrates that are found in fruits, vegetables, whole grains, beans, and other seeds. These valuable sources of nutrients are digested slowly, so you get a steady supply of energy without causing a sharp rise in your blood sugar.

inflammation, part of the immune reaction that protects you from infection when you injure yourself. It causes redness, pain, and swelling. Inflammation can damage the inner lining of arteries and break off clots to block the flow of blood, which can cause strokes and heart attacks.

CRP levels fluctuate from day to day, and levels generally increase with age. CRP can be raised by any infection, high blood pressure, excessive alcohol, smoking, lack of physical activity, chronic fatigue, coffee, elevated triglycerides, insulin resistance, diabetes, sleep disturbances, depression, taking estrogen, or eating a high-protein diet. If you have none of these known causes, the best ways we know at this time to reduce CRP levels are exercise and a diet that includes omega-3 fatty acids. The statin drugs appear to protect against inflammation as well as high cholesterol, but they can cause muscle pain and other side effects and may keep you from exercising. Your CRP test result should be "negative" or "normal." If your CRP is elevated, try to correct the known causes listed above. (More on inflammation, infection, and heart attacks in Week 6.)

HOMOCYSTEINE

Homocysteine is a protein building block that accumulates in the blood-stream when your diet is deficient in the vitamins B-6, B-12, and folic acid. One of the functions of folic acid is to convert the essential amino acid methionine to the nonessential amino acid cysteine. Lack of folic acid blocks this reaction, causing an intermediate product called homocys-teine to accumulate in the bloodstream.

High levels of homocysteine increase your risk for heart attacks, strokes, and birth defects. Homocysteine damages arteries and forms plaque and clots. In 1994, the U.S. Congress legislated that folic acid be added to all commercial flour, and the heart attack rate has since gone down. However, you may still not be getting enough. If you find your homocysteine level is high, check with your doctor, get blood tests for folic acid and B-12, and eat lots more fruits, vegetables, and whole grains.

LP(A)

Lp(a) is a genetic disorder that causes clots to form and therefore is a cause of heart attacks, particularly in younger people (men under the age of 40 and women under the age of 60). Everyone with a family history of heart attacks in members who are young should get this test. If your Lp(a) is greater than 40, you may need to take the time-release form of the vita-min niacin at bedtime or after every meal, and in continually increasing doses, until your Lp(a) is below 40. Diet alone will not lower Lp(a) because the dose of niacin you need is much higher than you can get in food.

DASH Plus Fitness—Week 2: Pick Your Sports

Now that you've gotten your doctor's permission to begin an exercise program, let's get started. Pick any sport or activity that uses continuous motion (such as running, cycling, swimming, rowing, or dancing) that you think you might enjoy. Don't pick a sport that requires a lot of skill or strength that you do not have just to get started (in-line skating, rope jumping, or rock climbing), or one where an amateur spends most of the time standing around (tennis or golf). You can add this type of recreation to your program later, but for now, stick with a low-risk activity that you already know how to do or that is easy to learn. If you don't have any idea of what activity you might enjoy, start out with walking while you investigate other possibilities. The same principles apply no matter what activity you select (see page 251).

> ➤ **A NOTE FROM DR. GABE**
>
> Every aspect of your life will benefit when your body is in top condition.

GETTING STARTED

Start at a relaxed pace and continue until your muscles feel heavy and then stop. For the first several days or weeks you may be able to exercise for only a few minutes. If your muscles feel sore the next day, take the day off. Gradually increase the amount of time until you can exercise continuously for 30 minutes every day at a relaxed pace and not feel sore. You may progress rapidly to the 30-minute goal, or it may take you two, four, six weeks, or longer. No matter how long it takes, don't get discouraged. Taking on too much, too soon will set you up for injuries.

The best way to avoid an injury is knowing when to quit, and that's simple: if you feel pain, distress, or a "funny feeling," stop! Don't be a martyr. Out-of-shape muscles can easily become strained or torn. If you feel pain, or simply feel that something isn't right, stop for a minute, then try again. If you notice the same sensation right away, move on to another activity. But if the discomfort builds gradually, continue until you feel it, then rest. Alternate these short periods of activity and rest until you begin to strengthen your muscles and can do the activity continuously.

> ➤ **A NOTE FROM DR. GABE**
>
> In-line skating uses smooth motions so it would seem to be easy on your joints. However, arthritis researchers are concerned about joint damage from the vibration caused by skating on rough road surfaces.

ENDLESS CHOICES

Selecting a new sport or a piece of exercise equipment can be daunting because there are so many possibilities. Start today to investigate the resources that are readily available to you. If your office building or neighborhood has an exercise room or program, check it out and try the equipment. Ask your friends what they do. Visit a YMCA, commercial gym, community college, or any other nearby facility that offers classes or memberships. Make notes on everything that's available and what appeals to you. DON'T give in to high-pressure pitches to buy equipment or memberships until you know exactly what you want. Use the "Choosing an Activity for Fitness" checklist (page 251) to help you narrow down the choices.

ACTIVITIES FOR FITNESS
   Walking
   Jogging
   Running

Swimming

Cycling

Rowing

Ice skating

In-line skating

Dancing

Aerobic dancing

Step aerobics

Cross-country skiing

Racquetball

Handball

Squash

Spinning classes

AEROBIC EXERCISE EQUIPMENT CHOICES

Stationary bicycle

Recumbent stationary bicycle

Mini-trampoline

Treadmill

Rowing machine

Stair stepper

Cross-country ski machine

Elliptical trainer

BUYING EXERCISE EQUIPMENT

There are lots of advantages to having exercise equipment in your home. You can exercise whenever it's convenient, in any weather. You never have to wait in line. You have privacy—a real plus if you're embarrassed about your weight or lack of fitness. You can watch television or listen to music while you exercise.

But good exercise equipment can be expensive. Make sure you know just what you want before you buy. If you have access to a health club or gym, try out the equipment that interests you. It's best to work through the first several weeks of a new exercise program on someone else's machine just to make sure you're comfortable, can master the movements, and—hopefully—enjoy the activity. That way you're less likely to end up with an expensive clothes hanger.

Once you've settled on the type of machine you want, find a store that carries several different models on display so you can try them out. Remember that health clubs buy extremely heavy-duty equipment; many machines built for home use are lightweight and poorly constructed. If you buy a machine that rattles and shakes, doesn't move smoothly, or fails to give you the range of resistance you need, you won't enjoy your workout. You don't necessarily need to buy the most expensive machine—you can do without all the electronic gadgetry. But do buy the sturdiest, smoothest-operating model you can afford.

DEAR DIARY

I encourage all my patients to keep an exercise diary, and I recommend that you do the same. When you record your progress in your journal, you have a written record that is a positive reminder of the healthy changes you are making in your life. An exercise diary is a great way to:

- Make yourself accountable each day.
- Track changes and gauge improvements.
- Help your mind focus on your goals each and every day.
- See how changes were made so that you can maintain your progress (and even review what to do if you get off track).
- If you suffer an injury, you can go back to your diary to see if you can figure out what caused the problem.
- Share your success and strategies with others who need help.

My Top Pick for Safety: A Recumbent Stationary Bike

Sixty-five percent of people who start an exercise program drop out in the first six weeks because of an injury. Jogging and running are high-risk sports because your feet hit the ground with a force greater than twice your body weight. This force can injure muscles, joints, and bones. Cycling and swimming are safer because you pedal in a smooth rotary motion, and when you swim, the buoyancy of the water reduces forces on your muscles.

The safest and most comfortable way to pedal is on a recumbent stationary bicycle. On a conventional bike, the pedals are below you, so you perch on a narrow seat and put pressure on the nerves in your crotch. When you pedal a recumbent bike, your legs are above your pelvis, so you can sit in a chair that does not pinch nerves. You lean against the seat's back support, so it's comfortable for anyone with back problems. Even a 90-year-old with poor coordination and weak muscles can use and benefit from a recumbent bike. A person who has had a stroke can tie his weak leg to one pedal and do all the pushing with the stronger leg. Anyone who can sit in a chair can use a recumbent stationary bike.

Multiple Muscle-Group Machines

Don't bother looking for an exercise machine that stresses more than one group of muscles at the same time (for example, a stationary bicycle that also moves your arms). Your brain will make you concentrate on the muscles that are doing the most work (in this case, your thighs, which are moving the pedals), and the muscle groups that don't need to exert force will just go along for the ride. A better choice would be an ordinary stationary bicycle plus separate weight-training exercises that work your arms.

You can use a calendar with large date boxes, a pocket appointment diary, or a plain notebook. We've included a Fitness Log in the Worksheets section at the back of this book. If you're a high-tech person, use your PDA or computer. Many programs are available for fitness buffs, or you can set up your own. When you are starting a new exercise program, jot down the length of time you exercised and your distance. You may want to add comments for yourself (how hard you worked, whether you had any discomfort, etc.). Later you will want to record more detailed information.

Keeping a diary should NOT make you feel that you must exercise a certain amount or go a certain distance every day. Don't be afraid to take days off when you need them. Listen to your body and rest or go easy whenever you are sore. If you find that you need to take a lot of days off, you might want to add a second activity that uses a different set of muscles.

SUPPORT YOUR LOVED ONE

How can you get your spouse or other loved one to become more active if they're not the least bit motivated? It's always hard to get someone else to move from being a couch potato to a dynamo; the excuses are endless. But couples who exercise together have the lowest drop-out rates of all beginning exercisers. So find something you and your partner can do together, even if one of you is more fit than the other. It's ideal if you can find something that's fun for both of you, but if you can't, for now you should cater to the possible interests or whims of the one who's inactive. You can both go to an aerobic dance class even if you feel silly doing it. Then YOU take the initiative for everything: get the memberships or equipment, clear the schedule, find a babysitter, do the dishes; remove every possible obstacle you can think of. Then go! Coach your loved one using all the techniques we've discussed for starting a new exercise program gradually. And be a cheerleader: "You're doing great!" "That color looks wonderful on you!" "That was a really hard move!" Or whatever nice things you can think of to say.

A Healthy Heart Does Not Hurt During Exercise

A healthy heart is so strong that it is not the cause of tiredness during exercise. Tiredness during exercise comes from your skeletal muscles when they run out of fuel or oxygen. Skeletal muscles use both fat and sugar for energy. When your muscles run out of their stored sugar supply, called glycogen, they cannot contract and function adequately. You feel tired, your muscles hurt, and you have difficulty coordinating them. On the other hand, your heart muscle gets energy directly from fat and sugar in your blood and even from a product of metabolism called lactic acid. It is virtually impossible for the heart muscle to run out of fuel unless you are starving to death.

A healthy heart should never run out of oxygen, either. Oxygen comes to the heart through arteries on its outside surface. If these arteries are not plugged up with plaque, they are large enough to supply all the oxygen that the heart can possibly need. However, plaque in your arteries can block the flow of blood. When the heart does not get enough blood, it will hurt and can start to beat irregularly. Exercise will not cause a healthy heart to hurt. IF YOU DEVELOP HEART PAIN DURING EXERCISE, SOMETHING IS WRONG AND YOU NEED TO CHECK WITH YOUR DOCTOR IMMEDIATELY.

The best activities for couples are those that have a social aspect—a health club, a class, or just a group of friends—because it makes the whole effort more fun and is more likely to inspire the inactive person. For one sport that's ideal for couples who have very different levels of fitness, see page 145 on tandem bicycles.

One major DON'T: Never buy a piece of exercise equipment as a surprise gift in an effort to inspire your non-exerciser. It will probably be taken as an insult and the equipment will just gather dust. Trying out and choosing exercise equipment should always involve the person who is going to use it. If it's a family investment, take everyone along when you shop.

DASH Plus Food—Week 2: The SHOW ME! Diet

Would you like to prove to yourself—AND TO YOUR DOC-TOR—that you can lower your blood pressure, cholesterol, and triglycerides with diet alone? Then take my challenge and follow the SHOW ME! Diet for the next two weeks. You must follow it strictly—NO CHEATING. Then have your doctor repeat your blood tests and measure your blood pressure again. I think you will be surprised, even amazed, at how quickly you can change your test results, even if they are very high or if you are already taking medication. If you are overweight, you will probably find that you have lost several pounds as well.

After you have proven to yourself what diet can do for your heart health, you'll spend the next five weeks learning how to get the same results with a much wider variety of foods. I'll show you how to adapt my diet guidelines to your particular tastes and lifestyle.

I've already warned you that the only foods you will be eating on the SHOW ME! Diet are oatmeal for breakfast and whole-meal salads for lunch and dinner. But you won't need to go hungry, because you decide on the portion size. Don't stuff yourself; eat until you are comfortably full and satisfied. If you prefer frequent, small meals and snacks, that's fine, too; just divide up your salads and eat as often as you like. You can also have oatmeal at other times of the day if you wish.

WEEK 2 MENUS

The menu for every day of the next two weeks is exactly the same:

Breakfast: Oatmeal (fruit and milk optional, see below)
Lunch and Dinner: Mix and Match Salads (recipe on page 200)

BREAKFAST INSTRUCTIONS: Use a long-cooking oatmeal (rolled, steel cut, Scottish- or Irish-style oats). Do not use quick-cooking or instant types. To save time, cook a large batch—enough for several days or a week—following the package instructions. Store the leftovers in a refrigerator container, and reheat each day's portion in a microwave dish. Flavor your oatmeal with a little cinnamon or nutmeg, and add a handful of raisins or other dried fruit to the pot if you wish. You may also add fresh fruit—up to one cup—but you must eat the fruit WITH the oatmeal, not alone as a snack.

Note: If for some reason you cannot eat oatmeal, substitute brown rice or another whole grain flavored and served the same way as oatmeal. Look for brown rice with at least 3 grams of fiber. Or try Kashi Breakfast Pilaf, a mixture of whole grains that is delicious and widely available.

If you like milk on your oatmeal, use skim milk, nonfat yogurt, low-fat soy milk, or another vegetarian milk. Do not drink it as a beverage; this is for your oatmeal only. For breakfast, lunch, dinner, and any time

Take the SHOW ME! Challenge

If you're basically healthy but have a loved one who is in big trouble and not cooperative, challenge him or her to follow the two-week SHOW ME! Diet with you, and approach it as a competition. See whose numbers improve the most. No one will be hurt by two weeks of eating this way, and you may find you feel better, too. If you don't want to take all of the blood tests, just compare weight and blood pressures. (You can measure yourselves at no cost in most pharmacies.) If you both can make it through the two weeks and are impressed with the results, you'll have a solid basis for discussing the more long-term heart-health strategies of the 8-Week Plan.

Or get a group of people (from your office, health club, or family) to take the SHOW ME! Challenge together. Form a pool to see who can improve the most or who can most accurately guess their test results.

in between, beverages must contain NO calories. Use water (tap, bottled, sparkling, or flavored), tea, or any other calorie-free drink you like.

WHAT IF MY BLOOD TESTS ARE ALL NORMAL?

If you are satisfied with the results of your blood tests, you can skip the SHOW ME! Diet and go directly to Week 4 of the eating plan. However, lower is better, and even normal blood pressure, cholesterol, and triglyceride results can be improved with diet. And if your goals include some weight loss, two weeks of the SHOW ME! Diet will get you off to a good start. It's your decision.

Featured Recipes • Week 2 SHOW ME! Diet

Menu Plan • Week 2   See Weekly Menu Plan

WEEK 3

Blood Sugar, Insulin, and Refined Carbohydrates

If your triglycerides or HBA1C are high, your HDL is low, you store fat primarily in your belly or you are overweight, pay particular attention to this chapter.

If your triglycerides, HBA1C, and HDL are normal, the information in this chapter will help you control your weight and keep your risk for diabetes and heart attacks low for the rest of your life.

The minute Sally L. walked into my office, I knew she was probably a diabetic and was headed for a heart attack. How could I tell just by looking at her? She had a huge belly and very small buttocks. Sure enough, her lab tests showed triglycerides at 390, an LDL of 165, an HDL of 30, and an HBA1C of 9.8. I immediately put her on Glucophage™, sent her to Diana's cooking classes, and got her interested in riding a tandem bicycle with her husband. She lost 45 pounds in six months. Now she is not taking any drugs, her HBA1C is a normal 5.7, and she has every reason to expect a long, healthy life.

In Victorian times a large belly was a sign of prosperity and manliness, but now we know that having a lot of fat in your belly area increases your risk for heart attacks and diabetes. People who store fat primarily underneath the skin in their belly region also store a lot of fat around their intestines and in their livers, and it is dangerous to the heart to store a lot of fat in the liver.

When you eat, your blood-sugar level rises. The higher it rises, the more insulin your pancreas releases to keep your blood-sugar level from rising even higher. As soon as insulin does its job of lowering high blood-sugar levels, it is removed from the bloodstream by the cells in your liver. However, fat in the liver prevents liver cells from removing insulin from the bloodstream. People who store fat primarily around their bellies also store a lot of fat in their livers, which prevents the liver from removing insulin, which causes very high and prolonged blood levels of insulin.

You need insulin to prevent blood-sugar levels from rising too high, but too much insulin constricts arteries, which can cause heart attacks. Too much insulin also acts on the brain to make you hungry. It acts on the liver, causing it to make more fat. It also causes the extra fat to be deposited in the liver, abdomen, and underneath the skin around your belly, so you develop a beer belly. Extra fat in the liver causes a condition called fatty liver, which eventually can send you into liver failure and kill you. So storing fat primarily in your belly area increases your chances of suffering from a heart attack, diabetes, and obesity.

INSULIN RESISTANCE

Cells are like little balloons full of fluid. On the surface of each cell are small hair-like structures called insulin receptors. Before insulin can drive sugar into cells, it must bind to these insulin receptors. Insulin resistance occurs when many of these receptors are blocked so insulin cannot do its job. This is called insulin resistance. If the sugar cannot get into your cells, the amount of sugar in your bloodstream increases, causing a higher than normal rise in blood sugar after you eat. If the sugar in your bloodstream cannot get into cells it sticks on the cell membranes, where it is converted to sorbitol, which damages cells. This is the process that causes most of the nerve damage and organ damage in diabetics, which can lead to heart attacks, strokes, blindness, deafness, kidney damage, impotence, and amputations.

Resting blood-sugar level is around 100. Blood-sugar level should not rise higher than 160 after meals. If blood sugar rises above normal levels, the liver converts the extra blood sugar to triglycerides, hence high blood levels of triglycerides. These high triglyceride levels can thicken your blood and form clots, so HDL cholesterol in your bloodstream carries the triglycerides to your liver to remove them. This uses up HDL cholesterol, so HDL levels go down. As your blood levels of sugar continue to rise, your pancreas releases even more insulin to try to escort the sugar into your cells. As increasing numbers of your insulin receptors are blocked, you become diabetic.

SYNDROME X, OR LOW HDL/HIGH TRIGLYCERIDE SYNDROME

Until thirty years ago, most doctors felt that insulin was a good hormone and the more you had, the healthier you were. Then Gerald Reaven of Stanford University showed that people with high insulin levels are at high risk for heart attacks because insulin constricts arteries, including those leading to the heart. He coined the term Syndrome X to describe a cluster of symptoms that occur together in both men and women. If you store fat around your belly, have low blood levels of HDL, the good cholesterol, and high triglycerides, you suffer from Syndrome X and are at high risk for a heart attack. Many people (women as well as men) who suffer from Syndrome X have male-pattern baldness and a family history of diabetes. A woman with Syndrome X may also have Polycystic Ovary Syndrome (see page 45), with excess hair on the face and body, acne, large muscles and bones, and other signs of high testosterone levels.

The cause of all these abnormal findings is insulin resistance, a higher-than-normal rise in blood sugar after you eat. People with Syndrome X may not be diabetic, but they are at high risk for developing full-blown diabetes.

For Women Only

If you are a woman who stores fat primarily in your belly area, has irregular periods, large bones and muscles, acne, extra hair on your face and body, hair loss on the top of your head, or are having difficulty getting pregnant you may have Polycystic Ovary Syndrome (PCOS). Check with your doctor immediately, because this condition increases your chances of suffering a heart attack and developing uterine cancer, and it can be cured simply by treating you as a diabetic. One out of twenty North American women suffer from PCOS. These women often have a family history of diabetes and will probably become diabetic if they are not treated. We have known about this condition for more than a hundred years, but only in the last few years have we found the cause and a cure.

A woman is born with about 4 million eggs in her ovaries. Each month after puberty, one egg ripens and is released by the ovary. Women whose eggs ripen but are not released have PCOS, caused by high insulin and male hormone levels. Glucophage™, Actos™, and Avandia™, diabetic drugs that reduce insulin levels, also lower blood levels of the male hormone testosterone in women. So does a diet that restricts bread, pasta, and other refined carbohydrates. Since many doctors are not aware of this condition, don't test for it, and don't know how to treat it, any woman who has these symptoms should ask to be checked for PCOS. You can be cured by changing your diet and taking Glucophage™ (metformin) and/or Actos™ or Avandia™.

For Men Only

Diabetes is one of the most common causes of impotence. See page 97.

ARE YOU PRE-DIABETIC?

If your HBA1C is normal but you store fat primarily in your belly, take the warning that you are likely to become diabetic if you don't change your diet and exercise more. The "Inch of Pinch" test and Waist/Hip Ratio (see pages 11–12) tell you whether you should be concerned. High blood levels of triglycerides and low levels of HDL cholesterol also predict that you are on the road to full-blown diabetes.

High blood levels of insulin constrict arteries and raise blood pressure, so many people who have high blood pressure are also pre-diabetic. People with insulin resistance have an increase in small, dense, low-density lipoprotein (LDL) cholesterol, which is more likely to cause heart attacks than the large, buoyant regular LDL cholesterol. High levels of insulin also cause clotting, which increases your risk for heart attacks.

If you heed these warning signs and make the lifestyle changes now, you can avoid becoming diabetic. It's much easier to prevent diabetes than to reverse it, and the diet and exercise recommendations are the same: Avoid all refined carbohydrates; lose weight if you are overweight; and maintain a regular, vigorous exercise program—for the rest of your life.

HEART HEALTH FOR DIABETICS

Abnormal HBA1C test results are a warning of diabetes out of control. If you are a diabetic and your HBA1C is under 6.1, be proud of yourself and of your doctor. You are doing everything right. A diabetic who stays tightly controlled has little more risk for the harmful effects of diabetes than a non-diabetic. On the other hand, if your HBA1C is over 6.1, you need to change your diet, exercise more, and talk to your doctor about adjusting your medications.

Diabetes should be tightly controlled with diet and exercise, as well as medication as long as you need it. You should learn how to avoid foods that spike the highest rise in blood sugar. You already know the problem: When you eat, blood sugar level rises. The higher it rises, the more sugar sticks on cells. Once stuck on a cell membrane, sugar can never detach itself. It is converted to a poison called sorbitol that damages the cell. This is the process that causes virtually all of the harmful effects of diabetes: heart attacks, strokes, impotence, blindness, deafness, amputations, kidney failure, burning foot syndrome, and other nerve damage.

DIET AND EXERCISE

You probably won't be surprised to learn that my diet recommendations are exactly the same for type I and type II diabetics, pre-diabetics, Syndrome X patients, women with Polycystic Ovary Syndrome, and anyone who stores fat primarily in his or her belly area. These people need to avoid refined carbohydrates—foods made with flour, white rice, milled corn, and all added sugars. They should also lose weight and participate in a regular, vigorous exercise program. Your doctor may prescribe medication if you cannot bring your test results into a normal range with diet and exercise alone.

Avoid the foods that cause your blood sugar to rise quickly. These include all types of flour products: bread, pasta, bagels, rolls, crackers, cookies, and pretzels; refined corn products and white rice; and all products with added sugar. Eat lots of vegetables, un-ground whole grains, beans, seeds, and nuts. Eat fruits and root vegetables (potatoes, carrots, and beets) only with other foods.

EXERCISE AND INSULIN

Regular exercise does more than just strengthen your heart muscle; it helps to prevent heart attacks by lowering insulin levels. Your muscles store sugar in the form of glycogen to be used for energy. If your muscles are full of glycogen, sugar in your bloodstream has nowhere to go, but if the glycogen in your muscles has been used up by exercise, the sugar in your bloodstream goes directly into your muscles. This keeps blood sugar levels from rising too high and triggering secretion of extra insulin.

High blood levels of insulin lower HDL cholesterol and raise triglycerides, but do not affect LDL cholesterol levels. Exercise does the opposite by lowering insulin levels. Even if you are not diabetic or otherwise concerned with high blood-sugar levels, you can benefit from a regular exercise program that lowers blood insulin levels.

SORBITOL IN FOODS

If you've seen sorbitol as an ingredient in candies, gum, or other "sugarless" foods, don't be alarmed. It *is* the same substance as the sorbitol that forms on cells and causes cell damage in diabetics, but if you *eat* it, it won't hurt you. Sorbitol is a sugar alcohol that cannot be absorbed through your intestines. When you eat foods containing sorbitol, it passes through your body undigested and never enters your bloodstream.

TYPE I AND TYPE II DIABETES

Diabetics are classified by whether or not they produce their own insulin. People who produce inadequate amounts of insulin are type I diabetics and must be given insulin. The vast majority of diabetics (90 percent or more) make plenty of insulin but do not respond to it. These are type II diabetics. If you have diabetes and do not know which type you are, get a blood test called C-peptide to determine if your body can make insulin.

If your C-peptide is greater than 1, you should not be placed on insulin because there are several newer drugs that are safer and more effective (see below). Diet and exercise recommendations are the same for both type I and type II diabetics. However, only type II diabetics can hope to get off all drugs by making these lifestyle changes. Exciting research is currently underway for type I diabetics that may soon make it possible for them to make their own insulin.

DRUGS FOR TREATMENT OF TYPE II DIABETES

There are two types of drug that are used to treat diabetes: those that lower blood sugar and raise insulin, and those that lower blood sugar and also lower insulin. The safest drugs are those that lower both insulin and sugar. Virtually all diabetics should be taking metformin (Glucophage™) before meals. It prevents blood-sugar levels from rising too high and causing sugar to stick to cells; it also has an excellent safety record. However, since metformin can cause liver damage if the blood becomes acidic, it should not be given to anyone with kidney damage. (Healthy kidneys control the acidity of the blood. Only a person with damaged kidneys is at significant risk for blood becoming acidic.) Eating a few bagels will produce such a high spike in blood sugar that metformin will not be effective, so it must be used *in addition to* avoiding foods that cause a steep rise in blood sugar. If HBA1C cannot be controlled with diet and metformin, your doctor will usually add Avandia™ or Actos™. These drugs, which are essentially the same, have in rare cases caused liver damage, so liver tests must be done monthly, at least for the first few months.

You should be seen monthly by your doctor and get either an HBA1C test (that measures blood-sugar control over two months) or fructosamine test (that measures your control over two weeks). Each time that your HBA1C is above normal, you need to be more strict with your diet, and your doctor should adjust your medication. I try to keep HBA1C under 6.1 in all of my diabetic patients. If your HBA1C is still not under control, you will need to take a drug that raises insulin levels. If that doesn't work, you will need to inject yourself with insulin.

HBA1C FOR DIABETIC CONTROL: WHY 6.1?

Some doctors tell their diabetic patients that an HBA1C of 7 or 8 is fine. That may be true if you are willing to stay on medication for the rest of your life and continue to have an increased risk for heart attacks, strokes, and the progressive damage caused by sugar stuck on cells. I want my patients to have higher goals, and you should have higher goals, too. HBA1C under 6.1 means that you are at extremely low risk for nerve damage. You *can* achieve this with diet, exercise, and properly adjusted medication. When you get to your ideal weight and are exercising regularly, your doctor can begin to reduce your medication. Hundreds of my patients are able to control their diabetes with diet and exercise alone, and are off all medications. Once your HBA1C is under 6.1 and you are not taking any drugs to keep it there, you are "cured"—as long as you follow your new eating and exercising habits for the rest of your life.

TRADE IN THE EXCHANGE DIET FOR DASH PLUS

The Exchange Diet and other diets designed for diabetics are based on tiny portion sizes (½ slice of bread, for example) or on the complicated counting of carbohydrates. These diets allow for bread, rolls, or pasta as long as you eat only a little bit. With the DASH Plus program you won't ever have to leave the table hungry, you don't need a calculator, and most important, you'll get better control of your blood sugar.

UNDERSTANDING CARBOHYDRATES

Carbohydrates are chains of sugar molecules lined in a row. They are found in all plants and in foods made from plants, such as bakery products and pastas. Carbohydrates can be a single sugar, two sugars bound together, or three or four sugars. Thousands of sugars bound together are called starch, and millions of sugars bound together so tightly that you cannot break them down are called fiber.

Only single sugars can pass from your intestines into your bloodstream. After you eat, food that contains starch enters your intestines, where enzymes knock off each end sugar molecule consecutively, rapidly, and continuously, and they are absorbed immediately. All simple sugars and starches that are broken down rapidly go into the bloodstream rapidly and cause a significant rise in blood sugar.

Resistant starches contain long chains of sugars that cannot release their end sugars, so they are not absorbed. They pass to the colon where bacteria convert them into fatty acids that help prevent colon cancer and heart attacks. That's why you want to eat carbohydrates that release their sugars slowly and restrict the amount of carbohydrates you eat that release sugars rapidly. The easier it is to break carbohydrates down into single sugars, the higher your blood-sugar level rises and the more insulin you produce.

The most healthful carbohydrates are those with fiber, which nature puts in whole grains, beans, nuts and other seeds, vegetables, and fruits. The most dangerous carbohydrates for diabetics and people who are trying to lose weight are foods made from refined carbohydrates that have had fiber removed: flour, white rice, milled corn, fruit juices, and all extracted sugars.

Whole seeds are tight capsules that release carbohydrates slowly. Instead of eating bread, white rice, or pasta, use whole grains such as barley, brown rice, wild rice, wheat berries, oats, or quinoa.

Root vegetables, such as potatoes and beets, contain stored sugar and starches that cause a steep rise in blood-sugar levels, but they contain so many healthful nutrients that you should include them as part of a healthful diet. Potatoes, carrots, and beets can be eaten safely with other foods to slow sugar absorption. For example, eating a potato with a piece of fish slows absorption of the sugars. The same applies to fruits. When you eat fruit with your breakfast cereal or in a vegetable salad, the sugar is absorbed more slowly. When you eat fruit alone, blood-sugar levels rise quickly.

The most healthful way to eat is to leave nature alone. Eat carbohydrates the way nature packages them, without first grinding them into tiny pieces or squeezing them into juices that remove the fiber.

How Refined Carbohydrates Harm Your Heart

Wherever carbohydrates are found in plants, you will also find the B vitamins. When you eat carbohydrates, enzymes in your intestines break them down into single sugars. Only single sugars can pass from your intestines into your bloodstream, where they can be used for energy, stored as sugar in your liver or muscles, or converted to fat. Many different chemical reactions then break down the sugar one step at a time to release energy. Each reaction must be started by an individual chemical called an enzyme. The B vitamins are parts of these enzymes that start the reactions that break sugar into energy.

If any of the B vitamins are not available, the conversion of carbohydrates to energy is slowed and the carbohydrates are more likely to be converted into fat, which:

- Raises blood levels of triglycerides.
- Uses up HDL, the good cholesterol, which lowers blood levels of HDL and increases risk for heart attacks.
- Is stored in fat cells, primarily around your abdomen.
- Helps form plaque in arteries, which makes them stiff and raises blood pressure.
- Blocks insulin receptors on cells so you cannot respond adequately to insulin. This causes you to produce more insulin, which makes you hungrier, makes you store more fat, and leads to diabetes in susceptible people.

When you eat carbohydrates that have been separated from the B vitamins, minerals, and perhaps other nutrients that have not yet been identified, you increase your risk for diabetes, obesity, heart attacks, and high blood pressure. We do not have enough dependable research to know if taking the B vitamins separately (in other foods or supplements) is as healthful as eating the B vitamins as they come in nature, paired directly with the carbohydrates in whole grains, seeds, vegetables, and fruits.

WHOLE GRAINS PREVENT DIABETES

A report from the Framingham study published in the *American Journal of Clinical Nutrition* showed that eating whole grains in place of bakery products and pasta lowers high cholesterol, lowers high blood pressure, reduces body weight, and lowers blood-insulin levels. When you eat foods made with flour, your blood sugar rises quickly. Whole grains are like capsules that release their contents very slowly. It takes about an hour to cook whole grains because of this tight capsule, and your body still has a difficult time breaking up the capsule, so they are very slow to digest. Whole grains help prevent diabetes and obesity because they keep insulin levels lower.

HEART ATTACK? CHECK FOR DIABETES

Have you already had a heart attack? If so, you should have your doctor check you for diabetes as well. A study from Sweden shows that many people discover they are diabetic only after they have had a heart attack. Researchers recorded blood-sugar levels in men who had suffered heart attacks and then did sugar-tolerance tests at the time of hospital discharge and then three months later. They found that 35 percent had diabetic sugar-tolerance tests at hospital discharge and 40 percent had impaired sugar-tolerance tests three months later. What that means is that 40 percent of people who have heart attacks are diabetic, even though they may

The Atkins Diet

The best-selling diet books of all time were written by the late Dr. Robert Atkins. His thesis was that restricting all carbohydrates helps people lose weight. Give him credit: When he started preaching that carbohydrates, rather than dietary fat, may be the main cause of diabetes and heart attacks, he took a lot of abuse. Time has shown that he is partially correct, but you cannot restrict all carbohydrates for long without paying a price.

Any diet that restricts calories will cause weight loss and lower cholesterol, so you can expect the Atkins diet to do this. But a diet low in plants restricts your intake of the vitamins, minerals, and phytochemicals you need to stay healthy and prevent heart attacks. You can follow Dr. Atkins's advice to avoid foods made with flour and sugar, but don't restrict other carbohydrates. Ironically, Dr. Atkins's last book, *Atkins for Life*, encourages readers to eat whole grains, fruit, vegetables, beans, nuts, and other seeds. His final diet recommendations are very similar to mine, but unfortunately, this sensible message has not received much media attention.

not know it. The patients who were undiagnosed diabetics also had a much higher rate of sudden death from heart attacks than those who were not diabetic.

DASH Plus Fitness—Week 3: Training Principles from Competitive Athletes

Exercise helps you to burn calories and build muscle. The more active you are and the more muscle mass you have, the more of your favorite foods you can eat. As your heart becomes stronger, you will have more endurance. Your skeletal muscles will become stronger and your physical capabilities will increase. If you have high blood pressure, exercise will help to lower it. You can also improve your blood levels of HDL cholesterol. As a bonus, exercise can help you feel better by increasing the levels of vital neurotransmitters that put you in a good mood.

> ➤ **A NOTE FROM DR. GABE**
>
> Blood pressure, cholesterol, and triglyceride changes occur quickly when you alter your diet. Other changes occur more slowly. It takes time to lose weight, build muscle, and increase endurance, but you will start to see results within a few weeks.

Any kind of exercise is better than no exercise at all, but for cardiovascular fitness, your exercise program should be aerobic, intense, and regular.

Aerobic—Exercise is aerobic when you get your heart pumping harder and your breath coming faster. You need to exercise continuously to strengthen your cardiovascular system.

Intense—You won't get much benefit if you just shuffle through your exercise. You'll need to work out with enough intensity to increase your heart rate.

Regular—Exercise at least three times a week. Five sessions a week, alternating hard and easy work outs, or alternating sports or activities to work different muscle groups, is even better.

IF YOU JUST STARTED YOUR EXERCISE PROGRAM LAST WEEK, you are still doing "background" work and may only be able to exercise for a few minutes before you tire or feel sore. However, you can learn good training principles and start to apply them. Every exerciser should understand the principle of "stress and recover" regardless of his or her goals and level of fitness. Each day, go slowly until you feel the slighest bit uncomfortable or your muscles start to hurt or feel heavy. Then stop. Most healthy people can build up to 30 minutes of daily easy exercise in fewer than six weeks. Once you reach that goal, you are ready to start training.

IF YOU'VE BEEN EXERCISING FOR MANY MONTHS OR YEARS, these training principles will help you get the most from your exercise program.

STRESS AND RECOVER

You will not improve in your fitness program if you do the same training regimen each day. Athletes train by working out hard on one day, feeling sore on the next, and not working out strenuously until their muscles stop feeling sore. Improvement comes from stressing and recovering. A hard workout causes your muscles to burn, which damages them. You feel sore the next day because of the damage and should work out lightly until the soreness disappears. When the muscles heal, they are stronger than they were before the hard workout. Then you work out vigorously again. If you work out hard before the soreness disappears, you place yourself at high risk for injury. So, no matter what your sport, work out intensely, which causes muscle soreness, and on the following days work out lightly or take time off until the soreness disappears.

As you continue to work out strenuously, only after the soreness disappears, you will become progressively stronger and faster and have greater endurance. Athletes in most sports train once or twice a day in their sports, but they do not exercise intensely more often than every 48 hours. Many older people need several days to recover from each intense workout.

There is a difference between the burn of muscles in training and the pain of an injury. The burn usually affects both sides of your body equally and disappears almost immediately after you stop exercising. The pain of an injury usually is worse on one side of your body, becomes more severe if you try to continue exercising, and does not go away after you stop exercising. If you feel an impending injury, stop and do not resume that activity until you can do it without pain.

How Muscles Get Stronger

Your muscles get stronger from stressing and recovering. On one day, you go out and exercise hard enough to make your muscles burn during exercise. The burning is a sign that you are damaging your muscles. On the next day, your muscles feel sore because they are damaged and need time to recover. It's called delayed-onset muscle soreness. You finish a workout and feel great; then you get up the next morning and your exercised muscles feel sore. Muscle biopsies taken on the day after hard exercise show bleeding and disruption of the z-band filaments that hold muscle fibers together as they slide over each other during a contraction. When they heal, they are stronger than before the damage occurred.

We don't know exactly how muscles become stronger, but the likely theory is that when the muscle fibers are damaged, other cells release chemicals called cytokines that cause inflammation characterized by soreness (pain), increased blood flow to the injured fibers (redness), and increased flow of fluid into the damaged area (swelling). The damaged muscle cells release tissue growth factors to heal the damaged muscle fibers. If you allow the muscle soreness to disappear before exercising intensely again, muscle fibers become larger and increase in number by splitting to form new fibers. If you do not wait until the soreness goes away, the fibers can be torn and you are injured.

MAKE IT FUN!

You're more likely to continue exercising for the rest of your life if you find an activity that you love. When you're just starting out, it may be hard to visualize how exercise could ever be fun, because right now it just seems like plain hard work. Trust me, as you increase your endurance, meet like-minded people, develop your skills, and start to surpass a few people—instead of always being the last, slowest, or least coordinated—you'll begin to see that exercise can be much more than a chore. Here are some tips for making your new exercise program more enjoyable.

ADD MUSIC. Music is what many people enjoy most about aerobic dancing or spinning classes. Moving to your favorite sound is more inspiring than silence. Almost any sport can be done to music. Caution: If you use a radio or CD player outdoors, make sure the earphones do not interfere with your safety. You always want to be able to hear what's going on around you.

ADD PEOPLE. Find an exercise partner or a class, go to a gym, or join a club. You'll find local clubs for almost every major sport or recreational activity. Get involved! You're more likely to continue your program if it's a sociable time and other people count on your participation.

GO PLACES. Exercise indoors when you must, but on beautiful days take your exercise outside and enjoy the scenery at the same time. Use your activity as an excuse to explore your local parks, monuments, historic spots, and natural beauty. Go on a weekend tour or vacation with others who enjoy your sport. Or just breathe the fresh air in your backyard.

BECOME AN EXPERT. Whatever activity you pick, you'll enjoy it more if you learn all about it—the latest fashions and equipment, who's who among the professional and amateur stars, and so forth. Search the Web for interesting sites and join a discussion forum. Every activity has its enthusiasts, and you'll be amazed at how friendly and helpful they are.

REWARD YOURSELF. When you finish a particularly vigorous session, get a massage. Sit in a whirlpool or sauna. Go out to lunch with your exercise partner (to a DASH Plus–friendly restaurant, see page 123). Set goals and when you reach them, reward yourself. Then record your successes in your fitness notebook.

➤ **A NOTE FROM DR. GABE**

PLAN ACTIVE VACATIONS: Take a walking tour instead of a bus tour. If you're in good shape and love your sport, seek out special vacation packages that feature cycling, walking, hiking, paddling, and so forth. Be honest with yourself about your abilities so you have fun, not misery. Watch out for cruises: Will you really use the ship's gym, or will you spend your whole trip at the 24-hour buffet?

WHY ALL DIABETICS SHOULD EXERCISE

When you eat, carbohydrates are broken down into sugar, which goes from your intestines into your bloodstream. Your body stores sugar only in muscles and in your liver. If your muscles are full of sugar, there is no outlet for blood-sugar levels, so your blood-sugar level may rise too high and cause cell destruction. On the other hand, if your muscles are empty of sugar, the extra sugar goes into your muscles and does not cause a spike in blood sugar. So diabetics should exercise before or after they eat, or at any other time of day, as often as possible. Alternate hard and easy days so you don't injure yourself.

WHEN IS THE BEST TIME TO EXERCISE?

Fit exercise into your daily schedule at whatever time works best for you. Some people will tell you that you'll burn more fat if you exercise just before you go to bed or when you first wake up, but there are no good data to support either of these notions. For many people, the best time is just before they need to concentrate or think clearly, because your body temperature remains elevated for four to six hours after you finish exercising, your heart pumps more blood, and you are more alert. But the bottom line is: The best time to exercise is the time when YOU WILL DO IT.

No Such Thing as Spot Reduction

Sit-ups are fine for strengthening your abdomen, but don't believe that they will get rid of a fat stomach. When you take in more calories than your body burns, you store them as fat. You store more than half the fat in your body under your skin and over your muscles. Exercising a muscle does not get rid of the fat surrounding it. If it did, tennis players would have less fat in the arm that holds the racket, but they don't.

DASH Plus Food—Week 3: Introducing the Whole Grains

This is your second week on the SHOW ME! Diet, so your meals will be exactly the same as last week. Eating the same foods every day can be boring, I know, but you only have a few more days to go. Make another trip to your supermarket and look for some new vegetables, nuts, or seasonings to vary your Mix and Match Salads.

Next week you will have a lot more foods to choose from. You'll find that WHOLE GRAINS are featured in many of my recipes. Even though you won't be cooking them this week, I'd like to explain how whole grains affect your blood sugar and your heart health, and why they should be a mainstay of your diet—particularly if you are a diabetic or pre-diabetic.

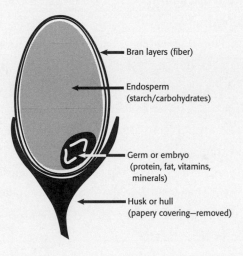

Whole grains are the seeds of grasses. The grass family is one of the largest and most abundant plant families on Earth, with more than 10,000 varieties. Grasses grow on all continents, including Antarctica, and have always been a major food source for the human race, as well as for many of the other animals who share our world. Whole grains were the first food humans learned to cultivate, making our transition from hunting-gathering to agricultural societies. The various grasses that grow in different parts of the world—rice, corn, wheat, rye, oats, quinoa, amaranth, and millet—became the "staff of life" for ancient societies. Grains are easy to grow and store, and they are excellent food, providing carbohydrates for energy, protein, essential fatty acids, vitamins, minerals, and fiber.

Our ancestors began to create nutritional problems when they found that they could store grains longer and could make them easier to prepare and more tasty by removing the parts that spoiled quickest and eating only the starchy part. They discarded the minerals, vitamins, phytochemicals, fiber, and omega-3 fatty acids that are found in the germ, creating serious deficiencies. We now have laws requiring that some of these nutrients be added back into commercial flours, but that has only corrected the most obvious problems.

Grains that are eaten as whole seeds are more filling and satisfying because they have more bulk and take longer to digest. Part of their bulk comes from water: Each seed swells when it cooks and soaks up water, which is carried in the grain until it is completely broken down in your digestive tract. (The water you drink, on the other hand, is absorbed directly from your stomach almost as soon as it gets there. Drinking water and other liquids will not "fill you up.") Processed grains absorb some water when you cook them, but less than the whole seeds, and the water is separated out more quickly during the digestive process. Most people can easily eat two or three cups of pasta, but you will find that you feel full with just a cup or less of whole grains.

Most important for diabetics, pre-diabetics, and anyone who wants to lose weight is that whole grains do not cause a sharp rise in blood sugar. The foods that cause rapid rise in blood sugar are those that are digested most quickly. The worst offenders are sugar and anything made from flour. When you eat whole grains, it takes a long time to break apart the seed capsule, separate the carbohydrates from the fiber, and completely digest each grain. Your blood sugar rises slowly, stays slightly elevated for a long time (so you don't feel hungry again soon after eating), and never reaches the high levels that occur when eating sugar or flour.

Whole grains will be the mainstay of your DASH Plus Diet. You've been enjoying oats, one of my favorite whole grains, for several days now. Next week I'll make sure you know where to find whole grains and how to cook them. Then you'll use them in some easy, delicious recipes: soups, salads, main dishes, side dishes, snacks, and even desserts. Your heart—and your waistline—will thank you.

> ➤ A NOTE FROM DR. GABE

Vegetarian DASH Plus is easy: Eliminate the seafood, use more servings of beans and legumes, and drink vegetarian milk substitutes. Be sure you have a source of B-12, which is found only in animals. Many vegetarian milks and cereals are fortified with it, or you can take generic B-12 pills.

DASH Plus Beverage Choices

When you exercise vigorously you can replace both calories and fluid with any drink you like. At other times, your beverages should not contain calories. If you drink juices, soft drinks, or milk to quench your thirst, you take in a lot of calories that do not fill you up. Eat your calories in food and quench your thirst with water or other calorie-free beverages.

Coffee or Tea?

Tea and coffee are made up of water plus phytochemicals, including caffeine, and very little else, unless you add a lot of sugar or cream. Both green and black teas come from the same plant, *camellia sinensis*. To make green tea, the leaves are steamed, rolled, and dried. For black tea, the leaves are dried, then fermented and fired.

Tea appears to be healthful and may contribute phytochemicals to your diet that you would not otherwise get. The same may be true of coffee, although it has received more bad press than good. Unfiltered (European-style) coffee can raise cholesterol, and caffeine can raise blood pressure. If caffeine makes you jittery, use decaffeinated tea or coffee. Enjoy one or two cups; what is beneficial in moderation may be harmful in large amounts. That's true for all foods, not just tea or coffee. If you want to drink more than a few cups of a beverage, make it water.

> ➤ A NOTE FROM DR. GABE
> **ALCOHOL HAS CALORIES, TOO.** If weight loss is
> one of your goals, don't forget to factor in the calories you get in
> alcoholic beverages: about 100 calories per 5-ounce glass of wine,
> 150 calories per 12 ounces of beer, 70 to 100 calories per one ounce
> of liquor. Don't believe the myth that your body burns these calories
> faster than other foods.

EXCESS MILK DEPLETES VITAMIN D

DASH Plus includes up to three cups of skim milk, cheese, or yogurt a day, or the equivalent in soy milk or other vegetarian milk substitutes. The dairy industry would like you to believe that drinking lots of milk is good for you, but researchers have shown that it's not a good idea to drink more than four glasses a day. The calcium in milk uses up vitamin D. Even though there is added vitamin D in milk, there is not enough to offset the loss of vitamin D caused by the calcium. So regular milk drinkers have lower blood levels of vitamin D than those who do not drink milk. Lack of vitamin D is a particular concern for people with dark skin and those who do not get outside in the sunshine often. Many studies link vitamin D deficiency with prostate cancer, particularly in African Americans.

JUICE IS NOT A HEALTH FOOD

An orange is more healthful than orange juice because it contains more than ten times as much fiber that helps to lower cholesterol, reduce weight, and prevent constipation. Juice raises blood-sugar levels more quickly than the whole fruit or vegetable because the fiber has been removed, leaving primarily sugar and water.

Diabetics and people who are trying to lose weight should not drink fruit juices because they contain the same amount of sugar as soft drinks and raise blood-sugar levels just as high. All sugared drinks are 6 to 10 percent sugar because that's the concentration that tastes best. Some fruits contain that much sugar, but juice makers add sugar to others. It makes no difference whether the juice is "100 percent fruit juice" or some mixture of fruit and sugar water. "All-fruit" juices often have added sugars

How Much Water Do You Need?

Your body needs fluid to function, but all foods contain water. Even the driest nut or seed has a lot of water in it. And all food is converted to energy, carbon dioxide, and WATER. Most people get the fluid their bodies need from food, and they need to drink only enough water to prevent constipation.

When you eat, the pyloric valve at the end of your stomach closes to keep food in. Then the stomach uses fluid that you drink and fluid from food that you eat to turn the solid food into a soupy liquid. If you don't drink enough fluid, your stomach takes fluid from your blood and adds it to the food in your stomach. The pyloric valve will not let food pass to the intestines until the food is liquefied. The liquid food passes to your intestines and then to your colon. There the fluid is absorbed to turn the liquid into solid waste. If you do not have enough fluid in your body, your body extracts extra fluid from your stool and turns its into hard rocklike pieces, causing constipation.

A reasonable amount for a healthy person to drink is one cup of water or any other fluid with each meal. If you have a problem with constipation, you may not be drinking enough water; but if you are not constipated, you are getting plenty. You'll also want to replace fluids whenever you sweat a lot, particularly in hot weather or when you exercise. Drink water whenever you feel thirsty, but there's no special health benefit gained from forcing yourself to drink eight glasses of water a day.

extracted from grapes, apples, or other fruits rather than from sugar cane. It makes no difference to your body whether the sugar came from the fruit or was added.

Eat plenty of whole fruits and vegetables, and drink juices if you can afford the extra calories and sugar. If you like juice, use a blender to make smoothies that contain the fiber or other nutrients not found in juices. Don't believe that juices give any special health benefits. Stick to water to quench your thirst.

SUGAR IS SUGAR

Don't push the sugar bowl away and replace it with honey, maple syrup, fructose, or any other sugar. As far as your body is concerned, there is no difference between honey and table sugar. Honey contains two simple sugars called glucose and fructose. Table sugar has the same two sugars, only they are bound together to form a double sugar called sucrose. In your body, they are processed exactly the same way. Once sucrose, the double sugar, reaches your intestines, it is broken down into the single sugars, glucose and fructose. It's the same with brown sugar, turbinado sugar, molasses, maple syrup, fructose, and so forth. When you need to be concerned about your blood sugar, it makes no difference whether extracted sugar comes from beets, sugar cane, flowers, apples, grapes, or maple trees. Avoid all sugars that have been extracted from any source.

WEEK 3 MENUS: (SAME AS LAST WEEK!)
  Breakfast: Oatmeal (fruit and milk optional)
  Lunch and Dinner: Mix and Match Salads

REMINDER: Arrange to get your blood pressure checked and your blood drawn at the end of this week. Ask your doctor to retest your cholesterol (LDL and HDL) and your triglycerides.

Featured Recipes • Week 3
SHOW ME! Diet

Menu Plan • Week 3

WEEK 4

Blood Pressure and the High-Plant (DASH) Diet

If your blood pressure is over 120/80, this chapter is critical for you.

If yours is normal now, this chapter will help you avoid being among the 90 percent of North Americans who will develop high blood pressure as they age.

Many people don't even realize they have high blood pressure, or hypertension. This "silent killer" can go unnoticed for years, quietly doing irreversible damage to your vital organs long before you know it's there. Some people don't find out they have high blood pressure until it's too late. That won't happen to you; you now know where you stand, and that you can lower your blood pressure with lifestyle changes.

You should be very proud of yourself if you completed your two weeks on my SHOW ME! Diet without cheating. Now it's payback time: Check your blood pressure again. Try to do it at about the same time of day and under the same conditions as the first check. Are you amazed at the improvement? Enter the results on your Before and After chart in the Worksheet section.

If you haven't already had your blood drawn to recheck your cholesterol and triglycerides, take care of that in the next day or two.

The way you have been eating for the last two weeks is a simplified version of the DASH Diet, which has been proven to lower blood pressure in 80 percent of people with hypertension. You can maintain the change in blood pressure, and the other improvements you will see when you get your blood test results back, if you follow the DASH Diet guidelines (with some modifications I'll explain below) permanently. No, I don't expect you to eat the same thing every day, as you have on the Show Me! Diet. In the remaining weeks of the 8-Week Plan, you'll build a repertoire of tasty meals using a wide variety of foods. You'll also learn how to follow my DASH Plus guidelines when you eat out, or if you think you're too busy to eat in a healthful way. If you are overweight, your blood pressure will continue to improve as you move toward your ideal weight.

Modified DASH Diet for Total Heart Health

A heart-healthy diet is a permanent change in lifestyle, not a short-term fix. The eating pattern I recommend is based on the DASH Diet, which is proven to lower blood pressure. However, I suggest some modifications to make the DASH Diet a diet for total heart health by further restricting saturated fats and refined grain products. I also suggest adding more beans (a good source of protein), and more sources of omega-3 fatty acids. The chart on page 70 compares the original DASH guidelines with my DASH Plus guidelines for total heart health.

These changes preserve all of the blood-pressure lowering features of the original DASH Diet, while adding other heart-health benefits. You already know why I stress whole grains instead of refined grain products. The other modifications reduce saturated fats and increase the "good" fats, which we'll talk about in Week 5. With these changes, the DASH Diet becomes the ideal diet for all of the common heart-health concerns.

But no diet, no matter how perfect, will build a healthy heart unless you also stay active, so my DASH Plus guidelines include exercise. DASH Plus guidelines should be strictly followed by anyone with diabetes, high cholesterol, and/or high blood pressure. For everyone else, the guidelines will offer a lifetime of good health choices.

Original DASH guidelines	DASH Plus guidelines
DAILY	**DAILY**
7 to 8 servings grains and grain products	About 8 servings WHOLE grains (no limit)
4 to 5 servings vegetables	At least 5 servings vegetables
4 to 5 servings fruits	At least 5 servings fruits
2 to 3 servings low-fat or fat-free dairy products	Up to 3 servings fat-free dairy products
1 to 2 servings meat, poultry, or fish	Up to 2 servings of seafood
4 to 5 servings per week nuts, seeds, or dry beans	Beans or legumes (no limit) Up to 2 servings nuts or seeds
2 to 3 teaspoons fats and oils	Up to 3 teaspoons olive oil (optional)
WEEKLY	**WEEKLY**
5 tablespoons of sugar, or its equivalent per week	Minimal added sugars MOST IMPORTANT—Exercise! DASH around!

The DASH study (Dietary Approaches to Stop Hypertension), supported by the National Heart, Lung, and Blood Institute (NHLBI) of the National Institutes of Health, was conducted at five sites: Brigham and Women's Hospital and Harvard Medical School, Johns Hopkins University, Pennington Biomedical Research Center, and Duke University Medical Center.

You'll be following DASH Plus for the rest of my 8-Week Plan. By the end of the program, I hope to have you convinced that this change in your eating habits is worth following for the rest of your life.

UNDERSTANDING BLOOD PRESSURE

You have two blood pressures: the systolic, which measures blood pressure when your heart contracts, and the much lower diastolic, which measures blood pressure when your heart relaxes. When your heart contracts, it pushes a huge amount of blood out to your arteries. Your arteries are supposed to act like balloons and expand to accept your blood and prevent your blood pressure from rising too high. Having plaque in your arteries stiffens them and prevents them from expanding when your heart contracts, causing your blood pressure to rise higher than normal. The stiffer your arteries, the higher your blood pressure rises.

Diastolic blood pressure is only a weak predictor of your susceptibility for a heart attack. The Framingham study shows that the systolic blood pressure is far more important than the diastolic blood pressure in determining your likelihood of suffering a heart attack or stroke. Your risk is

The Language of Blood Pressure

BLOOD PRESSURE is the force of blood against the walls of the artery.

HYPERTENSION is another word for high blood pressure.

SYSTOLIC PRESSURE is the highest pressure in an artery when your heart is pumping blood to your body.

DIASTOLIC PRESSURE is the lowest pressure in an artery when your heart is at rest.

Blood pressure measurement is made up of the systolic and the diastolic pressure. It is normally written like this: 120/80, with the systolic number first.

increased further if you have high blood cholesterol, sugar, or insulin; an enlarged heart; or if you are overweight. (The multi-million-dollar government-supported Framingham study, conducted by the Harvard School of Public Health, was started almost fifty years ago to see what lifestyle factors affect the health of Americans.)

WHY THE DASH DIET LOWERS BLOOD PRESSURE

Many studies show that the DASH Diet lowers high blood pressure at least as much as any combination of several drugs used to lower high blood pressure. Until recently, nobody really understood why the diet is such an effective treatment for high blood pressure. Now the DASH study team has shown that a diet based on vegetables, fruits, and low-fat dairy products acts as a natural diuretic that lowers people's blood pressure without drugs. The DASH Diet causes the body to urinate more salt in the same way that diuretics do.

Most people will not develop high blood pressure when they take in large amounts of salt because their bodies regulate salt concentration closely and they excrete or sweat out any excess. However, some people are salt-sensitive, and their blood pressures rise when they take in too much salt. Too much retained salt increases blood volume, which raises blood pressure. These salt-sensitive people benefit the most from the DASH Diet.

The DASH Diet is safer than drugs because diuretics can cause tiredness, inability to exercise, and impotence. A study in the medical journal *Hypertension* shows that the DASH Diet controls high blood pressure in people whose high blood pressure did not lower with an angiotensin receptor blocker. Those who benefited the most were African Americans who may suffer from an increased tendency to retain salt.

THE SALT SHAKER

Too much salt increases blood volume, which raises blood pressure. A plant-based diet, with few processed foods, is low in salt even if you sprinkle salt on your food. All animal tissues—meat, poultry, and dairy products—are full of salt. Most processed foods are high in salt even if they do not taste salty. For example, cookies often contain as much salt as potato chips. To prevent or treat high blood pressure with diet, reduce your intake of the natural food sources of salt: meat, chicken, whole-milk dairy products; and virtually all processed foods. These are the foods that also contain saturated fats, partially hydrogenated oils, and refined carbohydrates, as well as being low in antioxidants and other phytochemicals.

Whether you have high blood pressure or not, my advice is to go on my DASH Plus eating program, which includes lots of fruits, vegetables, whole grains, beans, and other seeds; start an exercise program; and add enough salt to your whole grains and vegetables to make them taste good. If you avoid most processed foods, as DASH Plus recommends, you will probably be taking in far less salt than you were before you started eating this way, even if you use a little salt when you prepare your vegetables, whole grains, and beans. Severe salt restriction is not healthful if you

Exercisers Need to Replace Salt

If you do not exercise, you do not sweat very much, and you do not need much salt; but severe salt restriction can cause high blood pressure, too. Exercisers can be harmed by salt restriction, just as some non-exercisers are harmed by taking in too much salt. If you don't have enough salt, your adrenal glands secrete huge amounts of aldosterone, and your kidneys secrete huge amounts of renin, both of which contract arteries and raise blood pressure. If you exercise vigorously, you sweat and lose a lot of salt, and low salt levels raise blood levels of aldosterone and renin. Furthermore, without the extra salt that you need, you will not recover from your hard bouts of exercise, and you will be more likely to get injured or feel tired all the time. Lack of salt is the most common cause of muscle cramps in exercisers.

exercise vigorously. It can cause muscle cramps, keep you from rehydrating properly, and may even RAISE blood pressure and cholesterol in some people.

WEIGHT LOSS, FIBER, AND BLOOD PRESSURE

The combination of excess weight and high blood pressure multiplies your risk for heart attacks and strokes. While the DASH Diet is not a weight-loss diet, most people who follow it lose weight because it limits dense sources of calories and fills you up with high-fiber fruits, vegetables, and grains.

The added fiber that you'll get from eating whole grains on the 8-Week Plan is also effective in reducing blood pressure. In one study on fiber and blood pressure, forty-six patients with blood pressures averaging 157/96 were given either tablets containing 7 grams of fiber or a placebo, which had no fiber. Three months later, the average blood pressure had dropped to 147/92 in the fiber group, but remained constant for those who took the placebo. These positive results were limited by the small amount of fiber the patients took in (only 7 grams a day) and the fact that it came in pill form, rather than from real food. Your results will be even better when you're eating more fiber in your food.

WHY BLOOD PRESSURE RISES WITH AGE

The National High Blood Pressure Education Program estimates that more than 50 million Americans have hypertension, but only about two-thirds of them have been diagnosed. Those numbers are likely to increase as our population gets older. An article from the Framingham study in the *Journal of the American Medical Association* showed that 90 percent of Americans will develop high blood pressure as they age.

The research shows that high blood pressure associated with aging is probably caused by damage to the arteries leading to the kidneys. This differs from high blood pressure caused by obesity or excess salt or alcohol intake, because high blood pressure from these causes is reversible. Taking in a large amount of salt, for example, can cause your body to retain fluid, enlarge blood volume, and raise blood pressure temporarily, but your blood pressure will return to normal soon afterward. The DASH Diet or diuretics reverse high blood pressure that is caused by salt sensitivity. Similarly, drinking alcohol raises blood pressure, but also only for a short time. And though obesity is associated with a sustained high blood pressure at any age, it is usually reversible with weight loss.

What researchers believe now is that damaged kidney arteries, called intimal fibroplasia, are the likely cause of the irreversible high blood pressure that occurs with age. Prevention of this type of high blood pressure includes preventing kidney arterial damage by eating plenty of fruits, vegetables, whole grains, beans, and nuts; reducing intake of processed foods and animal products; exercising; and keeping your weight down.

MEASURE YOUR OWN BLOOD PRESSURE

You don't have to wait for a doctor's appointment to measure your blood pressure. Many drugstores and supermarket pharmacies have blood-pressure check stations, which you can use at your convenience. If your blood pressure is an ongoing concern, you may want to invest in your own blood pressure cuff. Many different styles are available, but I recommend the digital wrist cuffs. Even though they are usually not as accurate as the arm cuffs, they are more convenient and easy to use. If you take your reading at the same time each day and under the same conditions, you will be able to monitor changes with reasonable accuracy. Keep your cuff in your bedside table and check your blood pressure first thing in the morning, before you get out of bed. Take three or four readings and, if they vary, record the average.

If your own blood pressure readings are consistently lower than those you get in your doctor's office, take your cuff along to your next appoint-

Drugs to Control Blood Pressure

If you cannot control your blood pressure with DASH Plus, your doctor may recommend adding drugs. If you are already taking medication for blood pressure, talk to your doctor about any side effects you may have and see if you can reduce your need for drugs as you lose weight and gain muscle.

Several recent studies show that the drugs of choice to treat high blood pressure for most North Americans are calcium channel blockers and angiotensin II receptor antagonists (ACE inhibitors). The American Heart Association recommends beta blockers and diuretics, but beta blockers can cause impotence, tiredness at rest and during exercise, and weight gain, and they increase your risk for diabetes. Diuretics make you tired. ACE inhibitors can make you cough.

Several studies have recommended different combinations of these drugs. The combination with the fewest side effects includes a calcium channel blocker and an angiotensin II receptor blocker. Long-acting calcium channel blockers relax blood vessels, while angiotensin II receptor blockers inhibit effects of a blood vessel-constricting hormone released by the kidneys. I start with angiotensin II receptor blockers and add a calcium channel blocker if necessary. If you're not sure what type of blood pressure medication you are taking, talk to your doctor or pharmacist.

Everyone on any blood pressure medication should follow the DASH Plus guidelines faithfully. It will help you keep the need for medication at a minimum and may help you get off drugs altogether.

ment and do an on-the-spot comparison. You may be a victim of white-coat hypertension, where your blood pressure rises just because you are with your doctor.

Resting Heart Rate

A slow pulse rate in athletes usually means a strong heart, but in non-athletes, it can mean heart damage.

Athletes often have pulse rates below 60 because their hearts are strong enough to pump large amounts of blood with each beat, and therefore don't have to beat as often. But non-athletes with slow heart rates often have damage to their electric conduction system. An electric impulse starts in the upper part of the heart and travels along nerves down the heart, causing the heart to contract and squeeze blood from its chambers to the rest of the body. If the nerves in the heart are damaged, electric impulses can be blocked and the heart can miss beats. This is called heart block and is a sign of heart damage.

Check your heart rate by counting your pulse for exactly one minute in the morning before you get out of bed. If you are an athlete with a slow heart rate, you are probably healthy, but if you do not exercise and have a pulse rate below 60, check with your doctor.

DASH Plus Fitness—Week 4: Your Heart Rate

IF YOU JUST STARTED YOUR EXERCISE PROGRAM, continue with your "background" work. Build up the amount of time you can exercise in each session at your own pace. Learn each week's exercise principles, but DO NOT apply them until you have developed enough strength and endurance to avoid injuring yourself. Record your progress in your Fitness Log.

IF YOU ARE AN EXPERIENCED EXERCISER, continue with your program. This week, learn to check your recovery pulse rate and make sure you are meeting your requirements for fluids and calories.

Many fitness experts suggest that you take your pulse during exercise so you can tell if you're working out at your target heart rate. But you don't need to do that because you can tell how fast your heart is beating just by paying attention to how you breathe.

The only heart rate that you need to know is the training heart rate that makes your heart stronger. To strengthen your heart, you have to exercise vigorously enough to increase your heart rate at least twenty beats a minute above your resting heart rate (see page 77). You can tell when your heart rate is high enough to strengthen your heart because your body will require more oxygen than it does at rest, and you will start to breathe deeply and more rapidly. You should feel comfortable and be able to talk. If you exercise so slowly that you never breathe deeply or rapidly, you are not strengthening your heart. On the other hand, you don't have to exercise as hard as you can to become fit.

MORE ON HEART RATE

An out-of-shape person and an in-shape person can exercise at the same heart rate, but the fit person will be able to do more work and move faster. The more fit you are, the more blood your heart will pump with each beat. So a marathon runner and a novice may both exercise at 140 beats per minute as they run around a track, but the marathon runner will go a lot faster.

EXERCISE AFTER EATING?

If you're in good shape, your mother probably lied when she told you not to go swimming after you eat. On the other hand, if you are in lousy shape, she was probably right. Your stomach is a muscular balloon that contracts and squeezes food into a soupy liquid before it passes into the intestines. Food in the stomach forces the muscles to contract, which requires your heart to pump blood to supply them with oxygen. When

Recovery Heart Rate

One of the best ways to measure your fitness is to check how long it takes for your heart to slow down after you've exercised vigorously. Hard exercise cannot hurt a healthy heart, but it can cause irregular heart beats in people who have damaged hearts. DO NOT USE THIS TEST UNLESS YOU ARE EXERCISING REGULARLY AND ARE SURE THAT YOU DO NOT HAVE ANY HEART DAMAGE.

Exercise in your sport as hard as you can for about ten minutes. Stop and immediately place your finger on the side of your neck where you feel a pulse. Count your pulse for only six seconds and multiply that number by ten to calculate your heart rate per minute. Do not count for more than six seconds because your heart begins to slow down immediately; you want a count that reflects your heart rate at your peak of exercise.

Wait exactly sixty seconds and then count your pulse for six seconds and multiply that number by ten. If your heart does not slow down at least thirty beats per minute in the first minute, you are in poor shape. If it slows down more than fifty beats in the first minute, you are in excellent shape. Check and record your recovery pulse rate periodically to measure improvements in your fitness.

you exercise vigorously, your heart must pump blood to your skeletal muscles. If you are in lousy shape, your heart may not be strong enough to pump large amounts of blood to both your stomach and exercising skeletal muscles at the same time, so the arteries leading to your stomach muscles close and your contracting stomach muscles do not get enough blood to meet their oxygen needs. Lactic acid then builds up in the stomach muscles and they start to hurt.

If you are in reasonable shape, your heart should be strong enough to pump blood to both your skeletal and stomach muscles at the same time. If you are going to exercise for more than an hour, you need to eat, or your muscles and liver will run out of sugar. Your brain gets almost all its energy from sugar in your bloodstream, but there is only enough sugar to last three minutes, so your liver has to constantly release sugar from its cells into your bloodstream. There is only enough sugar in your liver to last about an hour when you exercise vigorously. Eating before exercising can help you to exercise longer. If you do not eat before prolonged exercise, your liver can run out of its stored sugar, your blood-sugar level can drop, your brain then will lack its source of energy, and you will feel weak and tired. If you're in good shape, eat just before you exercise for more than an hour. If you plan to exercise more than two hours, you should eat and drink frequently during your exercise.

REPLACE FLUIDS AND SALT

When you exercise vigorously, you lose water through sweat. Sweat contains much less salt than blood does, so when you sweat you lose more water than salt, which causes blood levels of salt to rise. You feel thirsty during exercise only when the concentration of salt in your blood rises high enough to stimulate brain cells called osmoreceptors. You have to lose more than two pints of water for the salt concentration in your blood to rise high enough to make you feel thirsty. By the time you feel thirst, it is too late to catch up on your fluid loss, and you will have to stop exercising. By then you are dehydrated and have already lost two to four pounds of fluid. You may become nauseated, get muscle cramps, or feel dizzy. If you ignore the warning signs of dehydration, you can convulse and pass out.

When you exercise vigorously for more than an hour, you will need to replace both water and salt. If you exercise for more than two hours, you'll want additional calories, too. You don't need expensive sports drinks; use water or any beverage you like, and any food source of salt and calories.

Eating salt stimulates you to drink and raises your blood-salt level high enough to make you feel thirsty and able to retain fluid. Some sports drinks contain salt, but most people don't like the taste of a salty drink, so the salt content is usually too low to meet your needs for salt during heavy exercise. The potassium listed as an ingredient in some sports drinks is irrelevant, because you will not become potassium-deficient from exercise, plus you get plenty of potassium in virtually all foods.

If you need calories for vigorous exercise and prefer the taste of a sports drink over other beverages, use it. If your favorite beverage is cola, iced tea, lemonade, or water, that's what you should drink when you exercise, because you will drink more of the fluid you like best. Since your drink won't supply enough salt to meet your needs when you exercise for several hours, you'll also need to eat salted peanuts or anything else with salt that tastes good to you. For calories, it doesn't make much difference what you eat as long as the food doesn't remain too long in your stomach and make you uncomfortable.

Why You Sweat More When You Finish Exercising

More than 70 percent of the energy that powers your muscles is lost as heat, causing your body temperature to rise during exercise. To keep your body temperature from rising too high, your heart pumps the heat in your blood from your muscles to your skin, where you sweat it out, and the sweat evaporates to cool your body.

Sweating is controlled by the temperature of the blood flowing to the part of the brain called the hypothalamus. When your blood temperature rises, you sweat more. When you stop exercising, your heart immediately slows down, decreasing the amount of blood pumped to your skin, so the heat is not dissipated as rapidly and as a result your temperature rises higher and you sweat more.

When you're not exercising vigorously, don't get in the habit of using sports drinks or any other sugared drinks to quench thirst. They'll add up to a lot of calories with little other nutritional value. Drink water or a calorie-free beverage instead.

DASH Plus Food—Week 4: Two-Dish Meals

Y ou've been a good sport putting up with the same food every day for two weeks on the SHOW ME! Diet, and I hope you're pleased with the results. Now it's time to add variety to your meals. If you're an experienced cook, you can create your own menus using the DASH Plus guidelines below, any of the recipes in the Recipes section at the back of the book, or your own recipes that fit the guidelines.

If preparing your own healthful food is new to you, spend this week learning how to cook whole grains and start with a few of my easiest two-dish meals on this week's menu. While you're building a repertoire of favorite recipes, you can continue to use the Mix and Match Salads as often as you like. If you need to eat out frequently, see page 123.

> ➤ **A NOTE FROM DR. GABE**

If you like to snack, just divide your food into several small meals. This is better for weight loss than three large meals since you boost your metabolism every time you eat.

HOW TO COOK AND USE WHOLE GRAINS

Once you decide to add whole grains to your diet, you will find that you have lots of choices. All of the whole grains have bland, neutral flavors and can be used any way you would use pasta or white rice. You can add

DASH Plus Daily Guidelines with Serving Sizes

About 8 servings of whole grains (serving size: 1/2 cup; no limit).

At least 5 servings of vegetables* (serving size: 1 cup raw, 1/2 cup cooked).

At least 5 servings of fruits* (serving size: 1 cup raw, 1/2 cup cooked).

Up to 3 servings of fat-free dairy products or vegetarian milk products
(serving size: 1 cup milk or yogurt, 1 ounce grated cheese).

Up to 2 servings of seafood (serving size: 3 ounces).

Up to 2 servings of nuts or seeds (serving size: 2 tablespoons).

Beans or legumes (no limit).

Up to 3 teaspoons olive oil (optional).

Minimal added sugars; none if diabetic.

And MOST IMPORTANT—EXERCISE—DASH around!

Diabetics and anyone who is overweight should eat fruits and root vegetables (i.e., carrots and potatoes) only with other foods, not alone as snacks.

them to soups, top them with your favorite chili or pasta sauce, or mix them into salads. They are also delicious as hot breakfast cereals or as rice pudding–type desserts. Follow the cooking directions below and keep a variety of cooked whole grains on hand in your freezer, ready to make your own healthy "fast food." Most of the whole grains are interchangeable in recipes; use the ones you like or have on hand.

I always cook grains in bouillon or other flavored liquid. You can use bouillon cubes, granules, liquid, or paste. Make the required amount of liquid, following the directions for your brand of bouillon. Grains cooked in vegetable- or chicken-flavored bouillon will have a neutral flavor that can be used for any purpose: breakfast cereal, main dishes, salads, or desserts. If your bouillon does not contain salt, you may want to add a little to suit your taste. Whole grains cooked without any salt will taste flat to most people.

You do not need to rinse or pre-soak whole grains. The first time you cook a new kind, check them five to ten minutes before the end of the cooking time to make sure they are not getting mushy. If they aren't tender enough to suit you at the end of the recommended time, cook them a little longer.

Cooking Whole Grains in a Steamer

If you are serious about heart-healthy eating, get an electric countertop steamer. This is by far the easiest, most convenient way to cook whole grains. Look for one with at least an 8-cup capacity rice bucket and a 75-minute timer. Read the instruction booklet, then use the times and amounts shown in the chart below. Fill the steamer base with water to the top line. (Do not use the drip tray.) Place the steamer basket on the base. Place the grains and cooking liquid, such as bouillon, in the rice bowl and set it in the steamer basket. Cover it and set the timer. Let the grains sit for about twenty minutes after the timer rings before you remove the lid. You can let them sit for several hours if you prefer. This way you can cook

Steamer Cooking Directions for Whole Grains

FOR 2½ CUPS (1 LB.) GRAINS:	AMOUNT OF BOUILLON	COOKING TIMES
Wheat berries	4 cups	75 minutes
Whole oats	4 cups	75 minutes
Barley	4 cups	75 minutes
Brown rice	4 cups	65 to 75 minutes
Wild rice (½ lb.)	4 cups	75 minutes
Millet	4 cups	40 minutes
Quinoa	4 cups	30 minutes
Kasha (buckwheat)	4 cups	15 to 20 minutes

them while you sleep or go to work. Drain the grains in a colander if there is excess liquid.

COOKING WHOLE GRAINS ON THE STOVE TOP

Any of the whole grains can be cooked in a pot just as you would cook white rice, but they take longer and will use more liquid. Use a medium-size pot with a tight-fitting lid. Bring the liquid to a boil, stir in the grains, and return to a boil. Reduce the heat to low, cover the pot, and simmer until the grains are tender. Drain off any excess liquid.

Stove-Top Cooking Directions for Whole Grains

FOR 2½ CUPS (1 LB.) GRAINS:	AMOUNT OF BOUILLON	COOKING TIMES
Wheat berries	6 cups	60 minutes
Whole oats	6 cups	60 minutes
Barley	6 cups	60 minutes
Brown rice	5 cups	45 minutes
Wild rice (½ lb.)	6 cups	60 minutes
Millet	5 cups	20 minutes
Quinoa	5 cups	15 minutes
Kasha (buckwheat)	6 cups	15 minutes

OTHER COOKING METHODS

You can add raw grains to soups or stews while they cook, but it may be hard to get everything done at the same time without overcooking any of the ingredients. Some recipes use this method, but I recommend cooking the grains separately. Do whatever seems easiest for you. You can also use other appliances to cook whole grains; try what you have on hand.

RICE COOKER: If you have a rice cooker with a metal container and no timer, you may be able to use it to cook your whole grains, but you will need to experiment. These cookers use a sensor to determine when the liquid has been absorbed. Start with the quantities listed on the steamer cooking chart on page 84, and add more liquid if your grains come out too hard, less if they are too soft.

CROCK-POT: Add the quantity of grains and liquid listed on the stove-top cooking chart into your Crock-Pot or slow cooker, turn it on low, and leave it for six to eight hours.

PRESSURE COOKER: If you're comfortable using a pressure cooker, it will work just fine for whole grains. Refer to the stove-top cooking chart and adjust the cooking times as you would for any other food, usually about half the stated time.

FINDING AND STORING WHOLE GRAINS

Most larger supermarkets carry wild rice, brown rice, and barley. Ask at the customer service counter if you need help finding them. Your supermarket may have a health food section with various other whole grains. (The selection varies widely from store to store and region to region.) You will probably need to go beyond your supermarket to find some of the less common whole grains, such as whole wheat berries or whole oats. Check the health-oriented food chains, health food stores, organic markets, specialty gourmet shops, and food co-ops in your area. You can also check our Web site, www.healthyheartmiracle.com, for links to suppliers.

If you plan to store grains for several months, use containers made of glass, metal, or hard plastic to avoid insects. They will keep even longer if you store them in your refrigerator or freezer. Cooked whole grains should be refrigerated and will keep about a week in a covered container. If you don't plan to use up the grains in a few days, put leftovers in portion-size freezer containers or plastic freezer bags and freeze them. They are ready to serve after a minute or two in the microwave.

TWO-DISH MEALS

After you've cooked your first batch of whole grains, you're ready to make some two-dish meals. A typical meal at our house is a bowl with some whole grains in the bottom, covered with a tasty chili, curry, or vegetable stew that combines lots of different flavors, textures, and colors. With a crispy green salad on the side, and perhaps some fruit, the meal is

How to Pick a Cold Breakfast Cereal

The mainstay of the DASH Plus breakfast is whole-grain cereal. If you prefer cold cereals, check the list of ingredients on your favorite brands. The FIRST ingredient should be a whole grain, not "milled corn," "white rice," or "wheat flour," which are refined grains. Then scan the entire list and if you see the words "partially hydrogenated," put the box back on the shelf. Partially hydrogenated oils, or "trans fats," are used in an alarming number of cereals, even the ones that are supposed to be "healthful" (see page 93).

Once you've eliminated all the brands made with refined grains and/or partially hydrogenated oils, check for added sugars (you want little or none) and fiber (you want a lot). The fiber content listed on the nutrition label can be confusing because it's based on serving size, and very light cereals, such as puffed wheat, show little fiber per serving, but are fine when you calculate a serving by weight. Cereals made from bran (the outer covering removed from whole grains) will have higher fiber content than cereals made from whole grains, which have the germ and starchy parts of the grains as well as the fiber, but they can be hard to digest. The list on page 179 gives you lots of options.

complete. This may seem strange if you are accustomed to separate courses or plates arranged with separate piles of meat, potatoes, and vegetables, but give it a try. The possibilities are endless.

BREAKFAST CHOICES

The 8-Week Plan menus list the same breakfast every day, because that's what I eat: whole grain cereal, plus optional milk and fruit. You can use oatmeal or any other hot cereal made from whole grains, or select cold cereals using the guidelines on page 87. Feel free to use other foods at breakfast from the DASH Plus food list if you like. Unfortunately, most of the traditional breakfast foods other than cereals are full of refined carbohydrates and saturated fats and are best avoided.

Featured Recipes • Week 4
Easy to Prepare

WEEK 5

Atherosclerosis, Fats, and Fiber

If your LDL cholesterol is high, or if you are overweight, pay particular attention to this chapter.

All of us should be aware of the fats we need and those that are best avoided, as well as of the importance of fiber in our diet.

For ten years, I told Larry King that he was a walking time bomb and should change his lifestyle before it was too late. At that time he was doing his radio show all night and worked around the clock. He smoked to stay alert and, of course, he ate a tremendous amount of junk food. His blood pressure was 150/100 and his total cholesterol was 280. He suffered chest pains that were severe enough to take him to a cardiologist, but since his electrocardiogram was normal, he didn't see any reason to change his ways. When he had a heart attack, I was the first person to see him in the emergency room. Now he eats the way I do, exercises regularly, has normal cholesterol and blood pressure, and never felt better. His heart attack saved his life.

ATHEROSCLEROSIS

Some people are not as lucky as Larry King and don't get a second chance. A heart attack has two components. First fatty plaque accumulates in your arteries over the years and the flow of blood slows to a trickle. Eventually a piece of plaque breaks off, travels further down the artery, and forms clots, which block the flow of blood. The clots, which might have passed through a wide-open artery, block the blood supply to a part of your heart muscle, depriving it of oxygen and causing it to die. The same mechanism causes strokes, with a clot blocking blood flow to some part of your brain. I'll explain more about clots in Week 6. This chapter explains how plaque is formed and how changing your lifestyle can help to get rid of any you have and prevent it in the future.

LIPOPROTEINS—LDL, HDL, AND VLDL

The function of lipoproteins in your body is complicated, but I hope this explanation will help you understand why **HDL** is *Healthy* and **LDL** is *Lousy*. Fat is carried in your bloodstream in little fatty balls coated with protein called lipoproteins: HDL, LDL, and VLDL. When you take in more calories than you need for immediate use, your liver converts all of the extra calories into a type of fat called triglyceride. It doesn't make any difference whether the source of the extra calories is carbohydrate, fat, or protein. Then your liver takes about 1,500 triglyceride molecules, combines them with a lesser number of cholesterol molecules, and covers them with a protein coat to form a lipoprotein ball called **Very Low Density Lipoprotein**, or **VLDL** cholesterol.

VLDL travels through your bloodstream, giving up triglyceride molecules continuously as a source of energy for your cells, until it contains mostly cholesterol molecules and very few triglyceride molecules. The ball is now called **Low Density Lipoprotein** or LDL cholesterol, which is thought to be harmless. However, if LDL is oxidized by chemical reactions to form oxidized LDL, it can create plaque in your arteries. Fruits, vegetables, and other sources of antioxidants help to prevent LDL from being converted to oxidized LDL.

LDL is removed from your bloodstream by your liver. If you have too much fat in your liver, it clogs the LDL receptors on your liver cells so they can't do their job of removing LDL. As a result, your blood levels of LDL increase and more plaque is deposited in your arteries, increasing your risk for a heart attack. When you decrease the amount of fat in your liver by losing weight and taking in fewer calories, the number of working LDL receptors increases and your blood levels of LDL go down.

The good cholesterol, HDL, is manufactured by various cells throughout your body. It carries cholesterol from your bloodstream to your liver where it can be removed, so HDL helps to prevent plaque formation. You need enough HDL to remove the amount of LDL in your body. A blood level of 40 HDL is enough to remove 100 LDL, and so forth. Compare your numbers with the chart on page 24 to see if you have enough HDL cholesterol to remove your LDL cholesterol.

EXCESS CALORIES AND ATHEROSCLEROSIS

Taking in more calories than you burn leads to plaque in arteries in susceptible people. Fats are the most concentrated sources of calories, so a diet to lower LDL cholesterol limits fats, particularly saturated fats and partially hydrogenated oils. You need some fat, but for most people it's hard not to eat too much of it. Fatty foods are everywhere because manufacturers know that fat makes food taste good. Too many calories in your diet translates into too much fat in your body and in your bloodstream.

Fats contain nine calories per gram, while carbohydrates and proteins contain just four calories per gram. So eating a pound of fat will give you twice as many calories as a pound of carbohydrates or protein. Even if you are trying to avoid fat to lose weight, any reasonably varied diet will include plenty of fat, because all cells in food (except refined sugar) contain some fat. A heart-healthy weight-loss diet has enough of the "good" fats to meet your body's needs and avoids the "bad" fats.

TYPES OF FAT

All foods contain a mixture of the three types of fat: saturated, polyunsaturated, and monounsaturated. There are no foods that contain only one type. The three forms of fat are present in our food in varying proportions and are classified by these proportions. For example:

Types of Fat in Foods

FOOD	% SATURATED FAT	% MONO-UNSATURATED FAT	% POLY-UNSATURATED FAT	CLASSIFIED AS
Meat	52	46	2	Saturated
Fish	50	40	10	Saturated
Butter	61	36	3	Saturated
Olive oil	12	81	7	Monounsaturated
Corn oil	11	31	58	Polyunsaturated
Almond oil	9	70	21	Monounsaturated

SATURATED FATS are solid at room temperature. When you take in more calories than your body needs, saturated fats raise cholesterol and increase risk for heart attacks. Unless you burn a large number of calories, limit or avoid saturated fats found in butter, meats, and high-fat dairy products. Regardless of your weight, everyone should try to avoid partially hydrogenated vegetable oils, which are similar to saturated fats and are found in margarine, cookies, crackers, and hundreds of other processed foods (see page 93). Several studies link these chemically altered vegetable oils to increased rates of heart attacks and cancers.

MONOUNSATURATED FATS are liquid at room temperature. They are found in all food sources of fats, but particularly rich sources include olives, almonds, and other seeds. Before LDL, the bad cholesterol, can form plaque in arteries, it must first be converted to oxidized LDL. Monounsaturated fats are thought to stabilize LDL cholesterol and make it less likely to form plaque in arteries. Recent studies suggest that the heart-health benefits of these fats may come from antioxidants and other phytochemicals that accompany the fats in seeds.

POLYUNSATURATED FATS are healthful as long as they are left in their natural state, which is liquid at room temperature, and not converted to the more solid partially hydrogenated fats. Polyunsaturated fats include the essential fatty acids (omega-3s and omega-6s), which your body cannot assemble from other fats, so you must get them in your food. Omega-6s are abundant in vegetable oils and processed foods and most people get plenty. Omega-3s are found only in whole grains, beans, nuts and other seeds, and in seafood. You may not get enough of these fatty acids unless you make a special effort to eat these foods. Omega-3s are the least stable of the fats (they turn rancid quickly when exposed to air, light, or heat), so they are not found in most processed foods. Omega-3s help to prevent clotting and inflammation, so they decrease your risk for heart attacks and strokes. I'll explain more about this in Weeks 6 and 7.

PARTIALLY HYDROGENATED OILS contain trans fats. Removing polyunsaturated fats from vegetables shortens their shelf life, so to keep them from turning rancid, they are processed with heat, which destroys the very unstable essential omega-3 fatty acids. Or even worse, they are converted into partially hydrogenated oils. Food manufacturers add hydrogen atoms to replace the unsaturated double bonds between carbons to create a very stable, more solid oil that is similar to saturated fat but has a different chemical structure. Partially hydrogenated oils appear to increase risk for heart attacks by lowering blood levels of HDL cholesterol, raising levels of LDL cholesterol and Lp(a), and blocking arachidonic acid to cause clotting. Partially hydrogenated fats also lower blood levels of the inflammation-reducing omega-3 fatty acids.

Partially hydrogenated oils are the principal fat in many prepared foods, such as French fries, doughnuts, frozen meals, cookies, and crackers. Some major food producers, such as FritoLay, Kraft, and McDonald's, are responding to public pressure to get trans fats out of our food supply, but they are still widely used. I believe that all of us should keep the intake of partially hydrogenated fats in our daily diet as close to zero as possible. For tips on how to avoid trans fats, see 106.

GET YOUR "GOOD FATS" IN FOOD

The best fats are those you eat IN parts of plants—whole grains, beans, nuts, and other seeds. When you eat corn, olives, wheat berries, soybeans, sunflower seeds, or peanuts instead of their extracted oils, you get not only the calories but all the fiber, vitamins, minerals, and phytochemicals nature packages with the fat. People who need to lower LDL cholesterol or lose weight should avoid all added fats (butter, margarine, oils, and processed foods made with any of these ingredients). My DASH Plus guidelines suggest using no more than 3 teaspoons of olive oil per day. You also need to limit portion sizes of nuts and snack seeds, which are packed with nutrients but are so tasty that it's hard to stop at a reasonable portion size of 2 tablespoons per day.

THE ROLE OF CHOLESTEROL-LOWERING DRUGS

You get the maximum cholesterol-lowering benefit within a week of any diet change. If your LDL cholesterol is high, I hope that your two weeks on my SHOW ME! Diet convinced you and your doctor that you CAN control your LDL cholesterol with lifestyle changes.

However, if you were not able to bring your cholesterol values to nor-

Olive Oil and Your Heart

Two recent studies explain how olive oil helps to prevent heart attacks. One showed that it contains phenolic compounds that lower fibrinogen, which forms clots and damages arteries, causing heart attacks. The other study showed that olive oil is loaded with the potent antioxidants caffeic acid and oleuropein. These reports should not encourage you to go out and add olive oil to everything that you eat. All fruits and vegetables are loaded with antioxidants that help prevent heart attacks. You should interpret these studies to encourage you to eat large amounts of fruits, vegetables, whole grains, beans, seeds, and nuts, so that you will benefit from the many different antioxidants, anti-clotting factors, and cholesterol-lowering factors that are found in all plants. If you can afford added calories, olive oil is a healthful choice for salad dressings and cooking.

mal, your doctor will probably recommend cholesterol-lowering drugs. These drugs should be used IN ADDITION to your diet and exercise programs, not in place of them. All of these drugs have side effects, so your goal is to take as little as possible. If you have a lot of weight to lose, you will see additional improvement in your cholesterol numbers as you get closer to your ideal weight.

People who have high blood levels of LDL cholesterol benefit most by taking drugs specifically designed to lower LDL, such as Crestor, Lipitor, Mevacor, Lescol, Pravachol, Welchol, and Zocor. People with high LDL cholesterol are sensitive to taking in too much fat and too many calories. Their diet should restrict saturated fats found in meat, chicken, and whole-milk dairy products, as well as partially hydrogenated fats found in many prepared foods, such as French fries, cookies, crackers, and many bakery products. They must also reduce their total intake of calories, which means they must not resort to "low-fat" foods that still contain lots of calories.

On the other hand, those who have low blood levels of HDL cholesterol are sensitive to eating too many calories and too many refined carbohydrates, and should be treated as if they are diabetic (see Week 3). So they must avoid refined carbohydrates and reduce total calories. They may also need to take drugs specifically designed to raise blood levels of HDL cholesterol and lower blood levels of triglycerides.

I usually treat patients who have a low HDL and high triglycerides with an inexpensive generic vitamin called niacin. However, large doses of this drug frequently cause itching and skin redness forty-five minutes after taking it, so a time-release form of niacin should be used. If you take it just before going to bed, the problem will occur while you sleep and may not bother you. If the problem continues, you can often prevent it by taking an adult aspirin once a day. Check with your doctor.

Cholesterol in Your Food

Cholesterol is manufactured by all animals, so it is found in meat, poultry, fish, eggs, and dairy products. It is not found in plants, but you can be on a no-cholesterol diet by being a complete vegetarian and still have your cholesterol go up if you take in more calories than you burn.

Your own liver manufactures more than 80 percent of the cholesterol in your bloodstream; less than 20 percent comes comes from your food. When you burn all of the calories you take in, your liver keeps the amount of cholesterol in your bloodstream stable. If you eat more cholesterol from animal products, your liver makes less, and when you eat less cholesterol, your liver makes more. However, if you take in more calories than you burn, all extra calories are converted by your liver into extra cholesterol and triglycerides. It makes no difference whether those extra calories come from animal products (with cholesterol) or vegetable products (with no cholesterol).

Impotence

More than 80 percent of all cases of impotence is caused by atherosclerosis or diabetes, which blocks arteries. You need open arteries and undamaged nerves to have an erection.

A study from the University of Pittsburgh School of Public Health shows that as men age, their blood levels of testosterone drop. Those whose testosterone levels drop the most are the ones with high blood pressure and high blood cholesterol and sugar levels. Atherosclerosis blocks arteries, as well as damages testicles and interferes with their ability to make the male hormone, testosterone.

Your doctor will do a workup for other causes of impotence, but the odds are overwhelming that it will be caused by blocked arteries or diabetes. You can turn to pills, as millions of other men do, but for your heart's sake, deal with the root cause. You can reverse both atherosclerosis and diabetes with DASH Plus.

FIBER FOR YOUR HEART AND MORE

Fiber is the structural material of plants and is found in all fruits, vegetables, whole grains, beans, nuts, and other seeds. It is a type of carbohydrate that your body cannot break down, so you can't absorb it. There are two types: soluble and insoluble. Insoluble fiber adds bulk to your stool and helps to prevent constipation. Soluble fiber binds to fat in the intestines and keeps some fat from being absorbed.

Insoluble fiber may help to prevent colon cancer by speeding cancer-causing agents through the digestive system. It helps with weight control because it binds to water, creating bulk, which makes you feel full. It can also help to control diabetes because it slows the rate at which your body absorbs glucose.

Soluble fiber has an added benefit. When you add more soluble fiber to your diet, it lowers blood levels of plaque-forming LDL cholesterol. Soluble fiber is degraded by bacteria in the colon to form short-chain fatty acids that are absorbed into the bloodstream and help to block the synthesis of cholesterol by the liver.

When you follow the DASH Plus program you will get plenty of fiber. Don't worry about whether you are getting soluble or insoluble fiber; you need both kinds, and both are found in fruits, vegetables, whole grains, and beans. The goal is 25 to 35 grams of fiber a day, but the average North American consumes only 11 grams. There's very little fiber in the typical diet of hamburgers, pizza, fried chicken, and soda. Foods made from animal products never have any fiber, and processed foods made from grains, vegetables, or fruit frequently have most of the fiber removed. Wheat berries, baked potatoes, apples, and oranges contain many times more fiber than bread, potato chips, apple jelly, or orange juice.

STAY CLOSE TO NATURE

Anyone who is trying to control high LDL cholesterol or lose weight should avoid fats that are solid at room temperature: the saturated fats found in butter, meats, and high-fat dairy products, and all foods made with partially hydrogenated vegetable oils. The best fats are those you eat IN parts of plants—whole grains, beans, nuts, and other seeds.

DASH Plus Fitness—Week 5: Warm Up, Cool Down, Stretch

When you are able to exercise continuously in your chosen sport for more than a few minutes at a time, start each session with a warm up and finish it with a cool-down. You may also want to do some stretching after you have warmed up or during breaks.

WARMING UP

Warming up before you exercise intensely helps to prevent injuries and can help you to jump higher, run faster, lift more, and throw farther. To warm up, jog in place, moving your arms and legs, or spend five to ten minutes doing your sport at a very slow pace.

You do not warm up to increase muscle temperature, because heating a muscle does not prevent injuries or make the muscle contract with more force. You warm up to cause more muscle fibers to contract at the same time. It's called recruitment. Muscles are made of millions of individual fibers. When you contract a muscle for the first time in a workout, you use fewer than 1 percent of your muscle fibers. The second time, you recruit more fibers, and you continue increasing the number of muscle fibers used in each contraction when working that muscle for several minutes. Usually you are warmed up when you start to sweat. Then when you contract more muscle fibers, there is less force on each individual fiber, which helps protect them from injury.

COOLING DOWN

You should not stop suddenly after running very fast or exercising intensely because it may cause you to pass out. During running, your leg muscles serve as a second heart. When your leg muscles contract, they push against nearby veins and squeeze blood toward your heart. If you exercise vigorously and stop suddenly, your leg muscles stop contracting, and blood can pool in your legs, therefore not enough blood flows to your brain and you can pass out. When you slow down gradually, you allow time for your heart to pump harder to make up for the loss of pumping by your legs. However, cooling down does not prevent muscle soreness, which is caused by a tearing of muscle fibers during exercise.

STRETCHING

There's no evidence that stretching prevents injuries, but stretching properly can make you a better athlete. You are likely to injure yourself if you stretch before you have warmed up or when your muscles are tired. If you're over 50, be extra careful because older muscles are less springy and more likely to tear.

Competitive athletes need to stretch to make muscles and tendons longer to generate a greater torque about the joints they use to lift, run, jump, or throw. Stretching should always be done after your muscles are warmed up. Warming up raises muscle temperature to make the muscles more pliable. Stretch no further than you can hold for a few seconds. Bouncing gives you a longer stretch, but can tear muscles. Only competitive athletes need to stretch further than they can hold for a few seconds.

EASY STRETCHES

Head-to-toe strength and flexibility help you achieve and maintain good balance. Three-time Olympian and coach Pat Connolly, founder of Exersage™, offers these tips for building flexibility to help you prevent falls, pulled muscles, and back problems.

A muscle should be strong throughout its whole range of motion. Learning to *relax* a muscle helps it stretch and increase its range. Whenever you stretch one muscle, its opposing muscle contracts. For example, when you make a fist and curl your hand up to your shoulder, your bicep (in front of your upper arm) is contracting and your tricep (in the back of your upper arm) is stretching. So when you stretch a muscle, be sure to

---

> ➤ A NOTE FROM DR. GABE

Never stretch a strained or injured muscle. Stretching should not hurt. If it does, STOP.

loosen or shake it gently after each stretch. Start with the stretches below; next week you'll add some easy muscle-strengthening moves.

HEAD AND NECK

1. Sit tall in a chair, hands resting relaxed on your lap. Take a deep breath and slowly exhale, letting your shoulders drop and completely relax. Repeat three times.
2. While holding your head up straight, place the palm of either hand on your forehead. Then gently press against your forehead creating resistance as you curl your chin down to your chest, forcing the front muscles of your neck to work a little harder. Repeat ten times.
3. Place your hand on the back of your head while your head is hanging forward, chin close to your chest. Then gently press down on your head creating resistance as you roll your head back as far as it will comfortably go. Repeat ten times.
4. Shrug your shoulders, then relax. Hold your arms out to the side at shoulder level and then make slow backward circles squeezing your shoulder blades together each time you roll your shoulders back. Repeat ten times.

These exercises can be done any time you feel tense or have a headache. You'll be surprised at the relief you'll feel after just a few minutes.

ARMS

1. Stand with your feet about a foot apart, and let your arms dangle by your sides. Shake your hands for 5 to 10 seconds, then swing your arms up over your head and down, keeping them relaxed. Repeat ten times with each arm.
2. Lift your right arm, with your elbow pointing up and your hand hanging behind your head. With your left hand grab your elbow and gently push back, stretching the back of your upper arm. Hold for about ten seconds, then reverse arms.

TORSO

1. Sit in a chair, spread your legs apart, fold your arms, and bend over as far as you can between your legs, gently bounce to the left, middle, and right. Repeat five times.
2. Place your left foot on your right knee. With your right hand gently press your left knee toward the floor until you feel the stretch in your hip and buttocks. Repeat five times, then reverse legs.
3. Lie on your back on the floor. Bend both knees, keeping both feet on the floor, and sit up or curl up as far as you can. Hold for a few seconds. Repeat as many times as you can up to twenty. After you do this, lie flat with your knees slightly bent and gently shake your stomach muscles with your hands.

BUTTOCKS AND LEGS

1. Stand up and shake your left leg gently, slightly in front, and let your foot dangle for about 5 to 10 seconds. Repeat with your right leg. This helps to get the blood flowing. Then test the flexibility of the backs of your legs by bending over while keeping your knees straight, and see how close to the floor you can reach with your hands. Make a mental note or use a ruler. Then, after shaking out your legs to relax them, squat down, as if sitting on a low chair. Place both hands on your legs just above your knees, palm down with your fingers on the inside of your thighs. Now push your hands down on your legs as hard as you can and slowly count to ten. Stand up, shake out your legs, and then test yourself again to see if you can get closer to the floor. You should see an improvement.
2. Hold on to the back of a chair with both hands and gently swing your left leg back and forth ten times across the front of your body, then repeat with your right leg. Keep your swinging leg relaxed and your supporting leg straight. Then holding on with just your right hand, swing your left leg front and back ten times. Repeat with the opposite leg.

3. Hold on to the back of a chair with both hands. Put your right foot forward and slightly bend your right knee while your left leg is straight behind you, then try to press your heel down to the floor. Hold the stretch for a count of fifteen and then, *most important*, gently shake your foot so that you loosen the calf muscle you just stretched. Repeat with the other leg.

4. Hold on to the back of a chair with both hands. Extend your right leg behind you, keeping your knee straight, and raise your right foot about 6 inches off the floor by squeezing your right buttock muscles. Repeat ten times, then switch legs.

If You Injure Yourself

In case you overdo it and injured yourself, keep this acronym in mind: RICE (Rest, Ice, Compression, and Elevation).

Rest—Immediately stop exercising and rest the part of your body that is injured.

Ice—Place a bag of ice or a chill pack wrapped in a towel on the affected area.

Compression—Wrap a bandage around the affected area but don't make it so tight that it is constricting.

Elevation—Raise the injured area above heart level. If your back is injured, lie down.

Ice the injured area for ten to fifteen minutes, then repeat once every hour for the next several hours. The most effective treatment for muscle injury is rest, so don't exercise the injured area until the pain is gone. When you start exercising that area again, begin slowly and easily, gradually building to your previous level of intensity and duration. If you feel any pain whatsoever, stop and don't exercise that area until the pain has disappeared.

FEET

1. Using a chair for balance, stand on one foot and rise up and down on the ball of your foot 20 times. Repeat with other foot. Shake out your foot after each set.
2. Sit on a chair and make circles with your left foot, first pointing and then flexing. Repeat with the other foot.
3. Hold your legs straight out in front of you, point your toes as hard as you can and count to five, then pull them back (flex) as far as you can and count to five. Repeat 10 times.

> ➤ **A NOTE FROM DR. GABE**
>
> I don't recommend wearing ankle weights or carrying weights in your hands while you walk, run, or dance. They interfere with your natural movements, slow you down, and don't provide enough resistance to give any real strengthening benefit.

DASH Plus Food—Week 5: The Good Fats

The foods you eat when you follow my DASH Plus eating guidelines contain plenty of monounsaturated and polyunsaturated fats the way nature packages them: in whole grains, beans, nuts, and other seeds. This week's menus focus on tasty sources of the essential omega-3 fatty acids, which can be scarce in the typical North American diet. Omega-3s are found in seeds and seafood. Unless you are a vegetarian, include a variety of fish and shellfish in your heart-healthy diet. Vegetarians should be sure to eat plenty of seeds; flaxseeds are a particularly rich source. Omega-3s are the least stable of the fats, quickly turning rancid when exposed to air, light, or heat, so they are not found in most processed foods.

SEAFOOD

Fish and shellfish are good sources of protein, minerals, vitamins, and the essential omega-3 fatty acids. Fish contains more polyunsaturated fats and less saturated fats than meat from animals that are raised on land (beef, pork, poultry, lamb). You can get all of the nutrients found in fish from other sources, so if you're a vegetarian, you're not missing anything essential—as long as you eat plenty of whole grains, beans, and other seeds.

The richest seafood sources of omega-3s are the fatty fish that live in cold, deep water: tuna, salmon, swordfish, sardines, herring, mackerel, and anchovies. Clams, crab, squid, shrimp, and other seafood also contain omega-3s. Fish and shellfish are easy to prepare and add lots of flavor to main dishes, salads, and soups. This week's menus include a few of my favorite seafood recipes.

One easy way to increase the amount of omega-3 fats in your diet is to eat canned fish two or three times a week. Canned tuna or salmon can be added to salads or eaten right out of the can. Sardines packed in mustard or tomato sauce make tasty snacks. Both canned salmon and canned sardines (with bones) are also good sources of calcium.

Mercury levels have raised concerns about the safety of some large species of fish. I recommend that you not eat large amounts of any single type of fish caught in one location. This is one more reason to eat a varied diet and not to eat too much of any single food. I also recommend that you avoid raw seafood; some fish contain parasites that are harmful to humans, but they are killed in the cooking process. If you are pregnant or nursing, check with your doctor for the latest recommendations.

NUTS AND SEEDS

All seeds are highly nutritious packages containing protein, minerals, vitamins, fiber, and phytochemicals (more about them in Week 7). Since they also contain an energy source—fat, carbohydrates, or both—for the baby plant, they are concentrated sources of calories. Nuts, corn, cottonseeds, peanuts, flaxseeds, pumpkin seeds, sunflower seeds, soybeans, and other "oil seeds" contain mostly "good" fats: polyunsaturated and mono-unsaturated. They include varying amounts of the essential omega-3 and omega-6 fatty acids.

The DASH Plus eating guidelines do not limit portions of whole grains or beans, but nuts and snack seeds should be limited to about two tablespoons per day. Watch out for nuts if you're trying to lose weight; they taste so good that it's difficult to stop at two tablespoons. A 12.5-ounce can of peanuts is 2,200 calories. It's easier to limit the portion size

How to Avoid Partially Hydrogenated Oils

The only way to eliminate partially hydrogenated fats (the source of trans fats) from your diet is to read the label of virtually every processed food you buy. Scan through the list of ingredients and if it contains the words "partially hydrogenated," put it back on the shelf. Or patronize markets and food chains such as Whole Foods that do not stock any products containing partially hydrogenated oils.

It's much harder when you eat out, because you have no way of telling what's going on in the kitchen. Fast-food restaurants and chains use a lot of pre-prepared (read "frozen") foods that they reheat for you. These are usually loaded with partially hydrogenated fats. You're safer at restaurants that pre-pare your food from scratch. Asian restaurants are good bets. Their food may not be low-fat, but they contain oils, not margarine or shortening. Most French or continental restaurants (read: expensive) use huge amounts of butter—better than trans fats but not great if you're trying to lose weight or control cholesterol. Italian, Greek, Spanish, and other Mediterranean restaurants tend to use olive oil, a healthier choice.

of seeds used for flavoring, such as sesame, poppy, caraway, cumin, or fennel; or those that have virtually no flavor, such as flaxseed.

Salted nuts are an ideal food to take along for prolonged, intense exercise, such as cycling or running. They're easy to carry and are a source of concentrated energy. In addition, the salt along with the fluid you drink with them, will keep you from getting dehydrated. That's just one more reason for vigorous exercise—you get to enjoy lots of nuts!

DASH PLUS COOKING METHODS

If you can boil water, you can make any of the recipes in the 8-Week Plan. They all use easy, healthful water-based cooking techniques.

STEAMING. Food is cooked in steam that rises off boiling or simmering water. Steaming is good for vegetables that take a short time to cook, such as asparagus. You can use a special steaming pot, which keeps the food out of the water, or an electric steamer, which is also particularly handy for cooking whole grains (see page 84).

SIMMERING. Food is cooked gently in water or bouillon. Beans, whole grains, and long-cooking vegetables are usually simmered. Generally, you start with enough liquid to cover the food, bring it to a boil, and then reduce the heat to a gentle simmer. The pot may be covered or uncovered.

WET SAUTÉING. Food is cooked quickly in a small amount of boiling liquid. Put 1/2 cup or so of liquid in the pot, bring it to a boil, add the vegetables, and stir frequently. Add more liquid if needed to keep the food from sticking to the pot. Wet sautéing is useful for softening onions, celery, or green peppers before adding other ingredients. You can also "stir-fry" quick-cooking vegetables using the wet-sauté technique.

You can use these cooking methods on the stove top, in a countertop steamer or other appliance, or in a microwave oven; the choice is yours.

You can also occasionally broil, grill, roast, or bake. Broiled fish is particularly tasty. When you broil without adding butter or other basting fats, check the food frequently so you don't overcook it and dry it out.

Featured Recipes • Week 5
Good Fats

Menu Plan • Week 5   See Weekly Menu Plans

WEEK 6

Inflammation, Infections, and Heart Attacks

Everyone needs to be aware of the increasing evidence of the relationship between inflammation and heart attacks, strokes, and circulation problems.

If your C-Reactive Protein (CRP), homocysteine, or triglycerides are high, or if you have any chronic infections, pay particular attention to this chapter.

A high C-Reactive Protein blood level increases your risk of suffering a heart attack or stroke even more than having a high LDL cholesterol. C-Reactive Protein (CRP) measures inflammation, part of the immune reaction that protects you from infection when you injure yourself. When germs enter your bloodstream, your body produces white blood cells and antibodies that help kill them. The white blood cells produce chemicals called cytokines that bring antibody-containing fluids to attach to the germs, which causes swelling. Other white blood cells gobble up the invader. The resulting reaction of redness, swelling, and pain is called inflammation. Inflammation is good because it helps to defend you against infection. However, if you allow the inflammation to continue, or if your body produces inflammation when you don't need it, swelling damages your tissues, and you may suffer heart attacks, strokes, and a variety of other health problems.

The fatty plaque buildup that lines blood vessels often becomes inflamed because your white blood cells attack your own tissue rather than just germs. Fat cells are also known to produce these inflammatory proteins. Inflammation is thought to weaken the fatty buildups, or plaque, making them more likely to burst. A piece of plaque can then lead to a clot that can choke off the blood flow and cause a heart attack.

One study found that people recovering from heart attacks who had high levels of white blood cells are less likely to survive the heart attack. Other studies show that people who are given antibiotics immediately after suffering a heart attack or severe chest pains have 40 percent fewer repeat attacks over the next year. These studies suggest that heart attacks can be prevented by preventing inflammation, which can be caused by gum disease, diabetes, overweight, lack of exercise, smoking, high blood-cholesterol levels, or any infection.

These studies also suggest that you should treat every chronic infection. The evidence is not strong that stomach infections caused by helicobacter cause heart attacks, or that we can prevent heart attacks by treating chronic lung infections, chronic urinary tract infections, or reactive arthritis. However, I am willing to bet that in the near future, you will be told that these and other infections increase your chances of having a heart attack, and the next step will be to show that treating these conditions helps to prevent heart attacks.

If you have burning on urination or urgency when your bladder is full, a feeling that you have to urinate all the time, or get up in the night to urinate, ask your doctor to check for a urinary tract infection. If you have wheezing and a chronic cough or shortness of breath, check for a lung infection. If you have belching or a burning sensation in your stomach, get an upper GI series X-ray and a blood test for helicobacter. If you have diarrhea, check for an intestinal infection. I give my patients IGG and IGM antibody blood tests for chlamydia and mycoplasma. If the results are high, I usually recommend taking 100 mg of doxycycline twice a day for at least three weeks. Most doctors will not do this because they feel that data aren't yet strong enough to warrant antibiotics as a protection against heart attacks. The statin drugs appear to protect against inflammation as well as cholesterol, but they can cause muscle pain and make exercising difficult. At this time the best ways we know to reduce C-Reactive Protein levels are exercise and a diet that includes plenty of omega-3 fatty acids and keeps a proper ratio of omega-3s to omega-6s.

Ratio of Omega-3s to Omega-6s

For most of the time humans have been on earth, we have eaten foods containing omega-6s and omega-3s in a ratio of about 2:1. However, over the last fifty years in North America, the ratio has changed from 2:1 to a range of 10:1 to 20:1. Our diet now includes huge amounts of oils that are extracted from plants and used for cooking or in prepared foods. These oils, such as corn oil, safflower oil, cottonseed oil, peanut oil, and soybean oil, are primarily omega-6s. We have decreased our intake of omega-3s, found primarily in whole grains, beans and other seeds, and seafood.

Omega-6 fatty acids form prostaglandins that increase inflammation, while the prostaglandins from omega-3s help to reduce inflammation. Eating too many omega-6s and too few omega-3s causes clots and constricts arteries to increase risk for heart attacks, increases swelling to worsen arthritis, and aggravates a common skin disease called psoriasis. It may block a person's ability to respond to insulin, causing high insulin and blood-sugar levels and obesity. To get your ratio of omega-6s to omega-3s back to a more healthful 2:1, eat seafood, whole grains, beans and other seeds, and reduce your intake of processed foods and foods cooked in vegetable oils.

Drink Wine to Prevent Heart Attacks?

Healthy people can have up to two drinks a day without harming themselves, but having more than that often means a person is an alcoholic. A drink is 12 ounces of beer, 5 ounces of wine, or two-thirds of a shot glass of 100-proof alcohol. I consider a person who cannot stop drinking after the second drink to be an alcoholic. Several studies appear to show that people who have no more than two drinks a day have fewer heart attacks than people who do not drink at all. The explanation usually offered is that alcoholic beverages contain antioxidants that help to prevent LDL cholesterol from being converted to oxidized LDL, which forms plaque in arteries. If you enjoy wine or other alcohol and do not exceed two drinks a day, you may get some heart-protective benefit. If you don't drink now, I don't recommend starting just because of studies—often supported by industry interest groups—that suggest alcohol prevents heart attacks. Excessive alcohol can raise CRP and cause a variety of health problems.

DIGESTIVE PROBLEMS AND INFECTIONS

From your mouth to your colon, your digestive tract is loaded with bacteria, which makes it a common site for a variety of infections or inflammations that can raise CRP and increase your risk for heart attacks. Other digestive problems, such as constipation and irritable bowel syndrome, are usually caused by a faulty diet and are corrected when you adopt the DASH Plus guidelines. Specific food intolerances can be corrected by avoiding certain foods; lactose (in milk) or gluten (in wheat, barley, and rye) cause problems for many people.

All of these digestive problems can cause inflammation, and they may keep you from getting the nutrients you need or from making good food choices. Some digestive problems are difficult to treat, while others are easy; but none should be ignored. The brief summaries below highlight some of the more common digestive problems. For more information, visit www.healthyheartmiracle.com or check with your doctor.

HELICOBACTER PYLORI OR H-PYLORI: If you have burning in your stomach or esophagus, frequent belching, or any other symptoms of stomach distress, ask your doctor to do a blood test for Helicobacter pylori, the most common cause of stomach ulcers. One week on antibiotics plus an antacid usually cures the problem. I treat my patients even if the test is negative because more than twenty-three other types of bacteria can also cause these symptoms. You'll find more information on Helicobacter at www.healthyheartmiracle.com.

GAS: Whenever you change your diet, particularly if you add foods that contain fiber, you are likely to have an increase in intestinal gas. When carbohydrates (fiber and resistant starches) are not broken down and absorbed in the intestines, they pass to the colon where bacteria ferment the carbohydrates, releasing gas. This is perfectly healthful and the problem will probably diminish as you build a colony of "friendly" bacteria in your colon. Add new foods gradually. If the problem persists, check with your doctor.

CONSTIPATION: Gas is usually not painful unless you are also constipated, with pockets of gas stretching your colon where the gas is trapped by hard stool. The contents of your intestines are liquid until they reach your colon, where water is absorbed and stool is formed. If you don't drink enough fluid or eat enough fiber, the stool rapidly turns into hard rocklike pieces. To correct this, avoid all foods made with flour; eat lots of fruit, vegetables, and whole grains; and drink plenty of water. If this does not help, check with your doctor. Constant use of laxatives can deprive you of essential nutrients.

GLUTEN INTOLERANCE: In some people gas, diarrhea, cramping, and failure to absorb nutrients are caused by gluten, which is found in wheat, barley, and rye. You can try avoiding these foods to see if your symptoms are relieved, or you can have your doctor do blood tests for celiac sprue. If you are gluten-intolerant, you should also be checked for nutritional deficiencies such as lack of vitamin B-12 and iron.

LACTOSE INTOLERANCE: Half of the world's people develop gas and cramping after drinking milk because they lack the intestinal enzyme that is necessary to break down the double sugar called lactose, which is found in milk. If lactose is not absorbed in the upper intestinal tract, bacteria ferment it in the colon, releasing gas. If you are lactose intolerant, you can avoid dairy products or buy the lactose-free milk, which is widely available.

IRRITABLE BOWEL SYNDROME, CROHN'S DISEASE, ULCER-ATIVE COLITIS, AND OTHER CHRONIC PROBLEMS: The term Irritable Bowel Syndrome is often used to describe alternating diarrhea and constipation, a condition that can be cured by following the dietary changes for constipation (above). However, if you have more serious digestive problems that are chronic and disabling, you need a complete workup to find the cause. Check with your doctor, who will probably refer you to a gastroenterologist. The inflammation these conditions cause can increase your risk for a heart attack.

GUM DISEASE AND HEART ATTACKS

A study from the University of North Carolina at Chapel Hill reported that heart attack patients are at very high risk for having periodontal disease, including infections in the gums, bones, and teeth. Eighty-five percent of the heart attack patients in the study had periodontal disease, compared to only 29 percent of the healthy subjects. People in this study who had the highest CRP levels had the most severe periodontal disease. If you have bleeding gums, go to your dentist and get treated with the appropriate antibiotics.

The Friendly Bacteria

When you eat, enzymes from your intestines, stomach, liver, and pancreas break down carbohydrates into their building blocks called sugars; proteins into amino acids; and fats into glycerol, fatty acids, and monoglycerides, which can be absorbed into your bloodstream. However, many plant foods contain undigestible starches that cannot be broken down into sugars, so they cannot be absorbed in the upper intestinal tract. When they reach the colon, bacteria ferment these undigestible starches to form other chemicals, including short-chain fatty acids that protect your intestinal lining from irritation and cancer, and are absorbed into your bloodstream to lower cholesterol and prevent heart attacks. Recent research shows that normal intestinal bacteria are so numerous that they make up about 95 percent of the total number of cells in the human body. They also help to prevent bad bacteria from infecting you and may help prevent intestinal diseases.

You can eat live-culture yogurt or take pills that contain beneficial bacteria, but the best way to assure that you have a large colony of friendly bacteria in your colon is to eat plenty of the foods they work to break down: whole grains, vegetables, and other plant parts.

STRONG MUSCLES FOR STRONG IMMUNITY

As you age, you lose your ability to kill germs because of lack of muscle. When germs get into your body, you must make white blood cells and proteins called antibodies to kill them. Antibodies and cells are made from protein, and the only place that you can store extra protein is in your muscles. When you have large muscles, you have a ready source of protein for making antibodies and cells. When you have small muscles, you have a very limited source of amino acids to make protein, so your immunity may be inadequate to kill germs.

> ➤ A NOTE FROM DR. GABE

Muscles are your immune system's reservoir of protein building blocks.

Aging does not cause muscles to get smaller; small muscles are caused by lack of exercise. When you exercise, your muscles are damaged and they take time to heal from each exercise session. This cycle of muscle damage and healing is what makes muscles stronger. However, as you age it takes increasingly longer to recover from exercise. So older people often get injured, get tired too soon, or feel sore too early, so they do less and

Bob R. had triple bypass surgery at age 60. I warned him this was only a short-term fix and if he didn't change his lifestyle, the next blockage would probably be his last. He had a new wife and really wanted to stick around, so he ate the way I told him to, and he and his wife started to walk around the block every day. They found that they enjoyed being outdoors and gradually built up to a five-mile walk every other day. Other walkers they met along the way encouraged them to join a local walking group. At first they were happy just to complete their events, but then the spirit of competition hit them. They learned as much as they could about this popular international sport, got lots of training tips from their new friends, and soon started winning medals in their age group. They traveled to other cities for races and then overseas for major events. Now each year they arrange their travel plans around the race schedule. When I last saw Bob and Mary, they were heading off to Japan for a race. He said, "If you told me twenty years ago that exercise would become the center of my life, I would have fallen down laughing." His cardiologist is as proud as I am of our 82-year-old success story.

less and eventually stop exercising altogether. But this doesn't have to happen to you. Intelligent training practices will help you build and retain muscle mass, keep up your immunity, and live longer and healthier.

DIETARY PROTEIN

Protein supplies the building blocks for your muscles and all of the other tissues and functions in your body. These building blocks, amino acids, are used to make new cells and all the enzymes and other chemicals your body requires. Your body uses twenty-two different amino acids, and nine of those must come from the food you eat. These are called the essential amino acids. Your body can make the remaining amino acids from the essential nine. Most people need between 50 and 75 grams of protein a day. Protein deficiency is virtually unheard of in North America, since any reasonably varied diet will give you plenty. Before you decide to follow a fad high-protein diet or take protein supplements, understand that your body cannot store excess protein. Any unused protein is burned for energy or stored as fat. Large amounts of excess protein may stress your kidneys and liver and leach calcium from your bones. On the other hand, the Framingham Osteoporosis Study showed that women who didn't get enough protein had severe bone loss over several years. So eating either too much protein or too little protein can contribute to osteoporosis.

Meat, fish, and dairy products are good sources of protein, because they contain all nine essential amino acids. However, meat and dairy products also are high in saturated fat, so the DASH Plus guidelines suggest using seafood and skim milk products and avoiding meat, unless you are a competitive athlete or young person who burns huge amounts of calories.

Most plants contain some but not all of the essential amino acids. Strict vegetarians can get all the amino acids they need from whole grains and beans. The beans may contain only seven of the essential nine, but the grains will supply the other two. You do not need to eat special com-

No Grains or Beans?

Some popular authors tell you that humans should not eat grains, beans, or starchy roots because our caveman ancestors did not have these foods. Dr. Richard Wrangham, an anthropologist at Harvard University, thinks they are wrong. Other anthropologists think that humans have been cooking for only 300,000 years, which is not long enough for major evolutionary changes such as tooth shape or digestive-tract size to occur. Dr. Wrangham proposes that our predecessors survived because they were able to cook almost 2 million years ago.

Many of the most abundant plants on earth cannot be digested by humans in their raw state. Cooking softens hard seeds, breaks down toxic and irritating substances in roots and leaves, and releases nutrients bound up in plant cells. Starchy foods, such as potatoes, whole grains, beans, and cassavas, have 75 to 100 percent more digestible calories when they are cooked than when eaten raw.

Since cooking allowed us to eat both plants and meat, as well as to get more calories from many plants than when they are eaten raw, we had access to more food than all other animals. As a result, we survived when our competitors could not. Access to calories that were not available to non-cooking animals may also explain why humans evolved larger brains, which allowed us to dominate our environment wherever we went. Dr. Wrangham thinks the ability to cook a wide variety of foods allowed humans to develop into upright social animals with small jaws, small guts, and large brains.

binations of food at each meal to get "complete protein." Just eat a variety of grains, beans, and other vegetarian choices each week.

You convert the protein you eat into muscle only by exercising against resistance. That's why I recommend including weight training in your fitness program. When you work out vigorously, eating extra protein afterward can help your muscles recover more quickly.

DASH Plus Fitness—Week 6: Weight Training for Stronger Muscles and a Stronger Heart

It's never too late to build muscle. I've already explained how strong skeletal muscles make your heart muscle strong and serve as your immune system's reservoir of protein building blocks. Good muscle tone also helps you maintain correct posture and balance, prevent osteoporosis, move with ease, and look terrific. Large muscles even help you lose weight and stay slim because they burn more calories than fat, even when you are not working out.

With age, many muscle fibers die off and are not replaced. To stay strong, you must strengthen and enlarge the remaining muscle fibers to avoid the weakness and frailty seen in so many elderly people. Many older people can't get out of a chair without using their hands because their thigh muscles are too weak.

Exercise alone does not build large muscles; if it did, marathon runners would have the biggest muscles. To build muscle strength and size, you must move against resistance, using your muscles to exert a force against a counter force. Free weights, exercise machines, or even your own body weight can provide resistance.

Now that your program of cycling, running, swimming, or other aerobic activity is under way, it's time to add a weight-training component to your fitness program. Start out by focusing on the muscles that are not being stressed in your aerobic sessions. For example, if you are running or cycling, which use primarily leg muscles, spend your weight-training sessions concentrating on your upper body.

When you're first starting a weight-training program, I recommend going to a gym that has a variety of equipment and a staff that is qualified to teach you how to use it. Later, when you have established a routine and know what type of equipment you prefer, you may choose to invest in your own equipment so you can work out at home.

> ➤ A NOTE FROM DR. GABE
>
> If you need guidance or inspiration in your new exercise program, give yourself a gift: Hire a personal trainer.

Your instructor or coach should stay with you throughout your first few sessions to make sure you are holding the equipment properly and executing each movement correctly.

Start out with one to three sets of 10 repetitions, using a weight you can lift ten times in a row without losing form. When that weight becomes easy to lift, move up to the next level. You build stronger muscles by working with increasingly heavier weights, not by doing more repetitions. Eight or ten exercises using different machines is plenty. Your entire weight-training session should last no more than ten to fifteen minutes, unless you spend a lot of time resting between sets.

Lifting heavy weights causes a significant temporary increase in blood pressure, so check with your doctor before beginning a weight-training program or increasing your existing routine.

> ➤ A NOTE FROM DR. GABE
>
> Lifting heavy weights can cause a dramatic temporary rise in blood pressure. This does not cause problems for a healthy heart, but can break weakened blood vessels or cause irregular heartbeats in a weak heart. Always get your doctor's approval.

GETTING STARTED WITH WEIGHTS

You can start a strength-training program at home without expensive equipment, following these suggestions from three-time Olympian, coach of world and Olympic champions, and founder of Exersage™ Pat Connolly. Add the exercises to the stretching routine you started last week, and you can improve your strength and flexibility in less than 20 minutes a day. Don't push yourself if any of these moves are difficult for you. Start small and build gradually.

You'll need a sturdy, straight-back chair, a small fanny pack full of loose change, and two half-gallon plastic milk containers with handles. Begin with the containers half full of water.

AFTER YOU HAVE DONE YOUR ARM STRETCHES

Hold one of the containers in your right hand with your arm down at your side. Curl the container up in front and then down, then lift it as far back as you can. Repeat ten times. Do the same with your left hand. As you get stronger you can increase the weight by adding more water, then increase the number of repetitions to twenty, and eventually increase to two to three sets of the exercise.

AFTER YOU HAVE DONE YOUR LEG STRETCHES

1. Hold a container in each hand with your arms down at your sides. Stand in front of the chair and squat down far enough to just touch the chair seat with your butt; then stand back up. Repeat 10 times. As this gets easy, increase the weight of the containers, put the weighted fanny pack around your waist, and build up to twenty repetitions.

2. Sit on the floor with your legs straight out in front of you and your back against a wall. Wrap the fanny pack around one ankle and keeping your knee straight, raise that leg 10 times. Repeat with the other leg.

MUSCLES DO NOT TURN INTO FAT

If you are afraid to lift weights because you think that after you stop your muscles will turn to fat, you are mistaken. When you exercise, your muscles become larger and stronger because exercise causes extra amino acids, or protein building blocks, to deposit in muscles. All day long, amino acids pass from your muscles into your bloodstream and then back into your muscles because of exercise. When you stop exercising, fewer amino acids go back into your muscles and the muscles become smaller. These extra amino acids are picked up by your liver. Since your body has no way to store extra protein, your liver uses the extra amino acids for energy or converts them into fat. If you stop exercising, you must also eat less or you will gain weight—but muscles never turn into fat.

STRONG MUSCLES MAKE STRONG BONES

When you build strong muscles, you also strengthen your bones. Almost all women and most men will get osteoporosis if they live long enough. If you break a hip from osteoporosis, you have a 20 percent chance of dying from complications within a year.

Just eating more calcium in your food or supplements will not make your bones stronger, even though lack of calcium in your diet can cause

How Exercise Lowers CRP

Nobody knows exactly how exercise lowers CRP (C-Reactive Protein), but one theory is that the vigorous flow of blood cleans arteries, sweeping bacteria from the artery linings and preventing inflammation. Vigorous exercise cannot hurt a healthy heart, but check with your doctor, because strenuous exercise could cause a heart attack if your heart is already damaged.

osteoporosis. You have to do something else to make your bones pick up the extra calcium. That's why it's so important for women to include weight training in their exercise programs, because exercise against resistance is the only non-drug stimulus we have for getting calcium into bones. If you already have osteoporosis, your doctor may recommend bone-strengthening medications as well.

Just exercising will not strengthen bones. Female marathon runners who do not eat enough food to meet their calorie requirements develop osteoporosis even when they run more than 100 miles per week. You can strengthen your bones by lifting weights at any age.

WALK STRONGER

Many older people walk slowly and with an unsteady gait and have such weak leg muscles that they can't get out of a chair without using their hands to push themselves up. If you are over 65 and would like to be able to walk longer and faster, start a leg-strengthening program. Machines are easier to use than free weights, and you are far less likely to get injured. You need to perform only two exercises: a leg press in which you sit in a chair and push a weight away from you with your feet along with a knee extension in which you straighten your knee against resistance. Three times a week, do both exercises 10 times, rest as long as you want, and then repeat each 10 more times.

DASH Plus Food—Week 6: DASH Plus–Friendly Restaurants

Following the DASH Plus guidelines doesn't mean you can no longer eat in a restaurant. For occasional meals out, use "The 19 Meals for Dr. Gabe Rule" (page 165). But if you have to eat in restaurants several times a week, there are lots of healthy choices. If you are working to control your weight, diabetes, cholesterol, or high blood pressure, you need to find ways to meet your special requirements.

- Find restaurants with large salad bars and load up on fresh vegetables and other goodies from the DASH Plus list. Order baked, broiled, steamed, or poached fish or shellfish for your entrée and ask to have it prepared with lemon juice instead of butter. Have steamed vegetables as an accompaniment and fresh fruit for dessert.
- Asian restaurants offer a wide array of tasty dishes with lots of vegetables and generous portions. Thai and Vietnamese restaurants and Mongolian grills are good choices if you stick to the vegetarian and seafood entrées, but make sure to avoid white rice. Explore other ethnic restaurants in your area, too, and see which ones offer choices that meet the DASH Plus guidelines.
- Your chances of finding whole grains in a restaurant are slim, but if you travel a lot, you might want to pack or shop for cereal to eat in your hotel. Large cities and college towns often have vegetarian restaurants that offer varied, flavorful meals made with vegetables, beans, and sometimes even whole grains.
- Don't eat bread, rolls, or chips while waiting for your main dish. Have them taken off the table.
- Start with soup. Tomato-based vegetable and seafood soups, such as Manhattan clam chowder, are good choices.
- Whatever you order, if the portion size is large, divide up the meal and ask to take the rest of it home. That way you'll have something for lunch or snacks the next day.
- Avoid most fast-food restaurants. Their food is loaded with fat and is very low in fiber. Some chains now offer salads, but they are often laden with chicken, cheese, and high-calorie dressings. Still, these are probably the best menu items if fast food is your only choice.

Here are some national chains that feature salad bars or offer enough vegetables to give you DASH Plus–friendly meals:

Applebee's
Black-Eyed Pea
Bob's Big Boy
Chili's
Denny's
Garden Fresh
Golden Corral
Long John Silver's
Lone Star Steakhouse and Saloon
Olive Garden
Ponderosa Steak House
Ruby Tuesday
Ryan's
TGI Friday's

MAKE YOUR OWN FAST FOOD

You'll notice that most of my recipes are made in a large pot and yield lots of servings. I do this on purpose so you can make your own fast food. Even if you have only one or two people in your household, don't cut the recipe in half or quarters. The meals will keep for several days in the refrigerator, and almost all of the cooked dishes freeze well. So make up a big pot of soup, chili, or curry. Refrigerate enough for a day or two of leftovers and divide the remainder into individual serving-size containers and stash them in your freezer.

The directions for cooking whole grains on pages 84–86 explain how to store the leftovers in freezer bags, so you will have them ready to reheat in the microwave. When you come home from work, all you need to do is heat some grains and one of your leftover main dishes. While they're heating, make a quick tossed salad and set the table. Put some grains in a bowl and top with chili, vegetable stew, or whatever else you have prepared. Dinner is ready in five minutes. That's faster than the drive-through at a restaurant.

Soon you'll be doubling the recipes and stocking your freezer. Be sure to label each container with the contents and date; they all look the same once they're frozen. Make sure to use up your supply within two or three months, unless you have a good refrigerator that doesn't cause freezer burn.

Salads that contain raw vegetables and fruits will not freeze well, but most of them will keep for several days in the refrigerator. They often taste even better the second day after the flavors have blended together. Leftover salads make good lunch choices because you can pack them in resealable plastic containers and carry them along in an insulated lunch bag.

Featured Recipes • Week 6
Make Your Own Fast Food

Menu Plan • Week 6   See Weekly Menu Plans

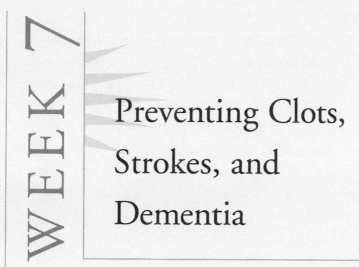

Preventing Clots, Strokes, and Dementia

If your Lp(a), homocysteine, or triglycerides test results are high, or if you have a family history of early heart attacks or strokes, this chapter is critical for you.

In this chapter everyone will find helpful tips for avoiding strokes, Alzheimer's disease, and other forms of dementia.

Your body is supposed to form clots only to protect you from bleeding, but any trauma or inflammation in your body can cause clots to form in blood vessels. If a clot breaks off from a blood-vessel wall, it can block an artery and cause a heart attack, stroke, or pulmonary embolism.

Clots can form wherever your body responds to injury or infection. When germs get into your body, they release chemicals that cause inflammation, characterized by redness, itching, swelling, heat, and clotting. Certain cells in your body, such as white blood cells and fat cells, also release chemicals that produce inflammation. Anything that damages tissue can cause inflammation, including trauma, burns, frostbite, irritants (such as corrosive chemicals), ultraviolet or other ionizing radiation, dying tissue from any cause (such as lack of oxygen during a heart attack), obesity, periodontal disease, smoking, excessive alcohol, gastroesophageal reflux (GERD), or allergic reactions.

Other factors that can lead to increased risk for clotting include genetic diseases such as Lp(a), dehydration, or blocked arteries or veins that can be caused by sitting in one position for a long time. Any clot has the potential to break off and cause damage, but you lessen your risk of blockage problems if your arteries are pliable and not already partially clogged with plaque.

KILLER CLOTS

While he was covering the recent war in Iraq, NBC reporter David Bloom died suddenly. A clot, which formed in his leg, broke loose from the vein and traveled in his bloodstream to his lungs, where it blocked the flow of blood. He had a pulmonary embolism, a deadly consequence of "Economy-Class Syndrome." When a person sits in a small space for a long time without moving, such as in a seat on an airplane, the knees are bent, which slows the flow of blood through the veins in the back of the legs, so that a clot can form in the deep veins of the calf muscles. David Bloom had been traveling in a vehicle whose interior was designed for safety, not comfort. He had reportedly been complaining of pains in his legs, a classic warning sign of a blood clot, or thromboembolism. The desert heat also caused dehydration, which thickened his blood and increased his risk for clots.

Embolisms of the kind that killed Bloom are responsible for an estimated 60,000 deaths in the United States each year. The underlying cause that makes people susceptible has been a mystery, but many experts believe that there is a genetic susceptibility to forming clots. Italian researcher Dr. Paolo Prandoni reports that clotting is linked to atherosclerosis, or hardening of the arteries, which leads to heart attack and stroke. Prandoni and his colleagues performed ultrasound examinations to take pictures of the carotid artery, the artery leading to the brain, in 299 patients with venous clots deep in their legs and in 150 healthy people. He found twice as much plaque, the fatty deposits of atherosclerosis, in the arteries of people who had suffered clots as compared to people who were healthy.

How to Avoid Economy-Class Syndrome

In Economy-Class Syndrome, a clot forms in the leg because it is bent for a long time without moving. This is a poor name for the condition because it has been reported in people sitting roomy first-class seats as well as in passengers sitting in the cheaper seats of an airplane. It is also a common occurrence on buses and cars, as well as in any place you have to sit still for a long time at work.

By now you know that you are at increased risk for heart attacks and strokes, as well as clots deep in your legs if you have high cholesterol, high blood pressure, store fat primarily around your belly, are overweight, do not exercise, eat too many refined carbohydrates and not enough vegetables, and so forth. When you are in an airplane or take a long drive or ride, stretch and move your legs frequently and, if possible, get up and walk around. You could save your life.

HOMOCYSTEINE AND LP(A)

If you are at high risk for heart attacks, you are also at increased risk for forming clots that can block the flow of blood, and disable—or even kill—you. Some people who have none of the obvious risk factors and are apparently healthy also are at high risk because of genetic factors or hidden dietary deficiencies that make them susceptible to forming clots. The most common of these are homocysteine and Lp(a), but there are others as well. People with a family history of heart attacks in younger years should ask their doctors to do a workup for possible causes of clotting. They will look for obesity, cancer, use of birth control pills, high cholesterol, or genetic conditions, such as factor V Leiden disease, that increase clotting risk.

Lack of any one of three vitamins causes the clot-forming homocysteine to accumulate in your bloodstream. You can lower blood levels of homocysteine to normal by taking folic acid, vitamin B-12, and pyridoxine. One of the functions of folic acid is to convert the essential amino acid methionine to the non-essential amino acid cysteine. Lack of folic acid blocks this reaction, causing an intermediate product called homocysteine to accumulate in the bloodstream. Homocysteine damages arteries and forms plaque and clots. In 1994 the U.S. Congress legislated that folic acid must be added to all commercial flour, and the heart-attack rate has since gone down. However, you may still not be getting enough. Folic acid is found everywhere in nature that carbohydrates are found, and it helps your body to convert carbohydrates to energy. You get folic acid from all whole grains and fortified cereals, leafy green vegetables, beans, seeds, nuts, and many other plants. You can reduce your intake of methionine by eating less meat. If you find your homocysteine level is high, check with your doctor and eat more fruits, vegetables, and whole grains. If you are a strict vegetarian or have low levels of vitamin B-12, you may also need to take supplements.

Several types of drugs used to prevent heart attacks have a side effect of raising blood levels of homocysteine, and therefore may actually increase risk for heart attacks. Anything that lowers blood levels of folic acid increases your risk for a heart attack. Metformin, which is used to treat diabetes, and cholestyramine, which is used to treat high triglycerides, block the absorption of folic acid from the intestines and raise blood levels of homocysteine. Likewise, niacin, which is used to treat high cholesterol and Lp(a), and methotrexate, which is used to treat arthritis, block the metabolism of folic acid in the body and lower blood levels of folic acid. If you are taking any of these drugs, you should eat lots of leafy greens and possibly take folic acid supplements as well. Your doctor can check your folic-acid levels with a blood test.

Lp(a) is a genetic disorder that increases your susceptability to clots. This hidden disorder is often the cause of heart attacks in young people (men under the age of 40 and women under the age of 60) who have none of the obvious risk factors. If your Lp(a) level is more than 40, the treatment of choice is niacin, taken in time-release capsules at bedtime or after meals. Your doctor will probably start with 500mg and continue raising the dose until your Lp(a) level is less than 40. Even though niacin is found in many of the foods in the DASH Plus plan, you cannot correct Lp(a) with diet, because the amount of niacin you need is too high to get from food alone.

EXERCISE IS THE BEST TREATMENT FOR VARICOSE VEINS

Veins contain valves that keep blood from backing up and pooling. When the valves cannot close properly, veins become varicose: blood backs up, causing the veins to widen and look like blue snakes underneath the skin. The best treatment is to empty blood from the veins with exercise. When you exercise, your leg muscles alternately contract and relax, squeezing blood back toward the heart. So running, walking, cycling, skiing, skating, or dancing are ideal activities, while standing or sitting increases blood pooling and widens your veins. Elevating the legs can help to relieve the pooling of blood caused by gravity.

Varicose veins can also be caused by a genetic weakness in the valves or an obstruction of blood flow caused by obesity, pregnancy, tumors, clots, or heart disease. Superficial varicose veins, which you can see, can cause a feeling of heaviness or aching, but they are rarely painful. Most varicose veins are best left alone. If you develop severe pain, usually in the veins in your calf muscles, you may have a clot and should immediately check with your doctor. Otherwise, exercise is the best medicine.

RUNNING DOES NOT CAUSE CLOTS

Dr. Art Siegel is a respected professor at Harvard Medical School and a former marathon runner. He published an article in the *American Journal of Cardiology* that shows that after a marathon, runners have extremely high blood levels of clotting and inflammatory factors associated with an increased risk for heart attacks. The media concluded from this study that running marathons can cause heart attacks.

Running damages muscles, and damaged muscles release chemicals such as CPK and von Willebrand factor, which cause clotting. Clots can block the flow of blood to the heart to cause heart attacks. Dr. Siegel showed that these clotting factors are released from muscles during a marathon. However, running also produces antifibrinogens, which prevent clotting. Furthermore, marathon runners seldom have plaque in their arteries, and we know that arteries narrowed by plaque are the most likely to be blocked by clots. The media should not have reported that Dr. Siegel's study showed that running marathons causes clots and heart attacks, because it doesn't.

STROKES, MINI-STROKES, AND DEMENTIA

All of the risk factors for heart attacks also increase your risk for a disabling stroke and—perhaps even more feared—frequent mini-strokes which deprive you of your memory and mental functioning, and Alzheimer's disease. One in ten North Americans has decreased mental function by age 65, and five in ten are affected by age 85. The lifestyle factors that increase your risk for Alzheimer's disease and other types of dementia are the same.

Recent research confirms that changing your diet and exercising more are the best ways we have to ward off memory loss. One study showed that people who have high blood levels of homocysteine are most likely to suffer Alzheimer's disease or dementia. To avoid this you should eat less meat and more leafy greens and vegetables. Another study showed that elderly people who eat seafood at least once a week are at low risk for becoming senile and developing Alzheimer's disease. A third study found that a diet high in the unsaturated, unhydrogenated fats that are found in plants may help lower risk. Another report from Columbia Medical School shows that people who develop Alzheimer's disease eat more food and fat than those who do not develop that disease. Following my 8-Week Plan won't guarantee that you'll keep your IQ intact, but it will greatly improve your chances.

B-12 DEFICIENCY AND MEMORY LOSS

Lack of vitamin B-12 is a common cause of senility. One study from Austria showed that B-12 deficiency may be missed by doctors because people with a deficiency often have normal blood levels of the vitamin. Many people suffer from vitamin B-12 deficiency because they have low blood levels of homotranscobalamine II, the protein that carries B-12 into your cells' mitochondria. So you can have normal levels of B-12 in your blood and not enough in your cells. When your body lacks B-12, your red blood cells do not mature properly and are much larger than normal, and homocysteine accumulates in your bloodstream. More dependable tests for B-12 deficiency are MCV, which measures the size of red blood cells; and a test that measures the blood levels of homocysteine. You only need about 2mcg of B-12 a day, but as people age they may lose their ability to absorb B-12 even when there is plenty in the food they eat. If you or your doctor are concerned about B-12 deficiency, almost everyone can absorb enough from inexpensive, generic 1000mcg B-12 pills that are available in any drugstore or supermarket.

PHYTOCHEMICALS FOR HEART HEALTH

All edible plants contain substances your body uses to stay healthy and ward off disease. In addition to vitamins and minerals, there are countless phytochemicals (phyto = plant, chemical = chemical) that help to reduce inflammation, keep blood thinned to the proper consistency, lower cholesterol and blood pressure, and perform dozens of other useful functions.

Plants use these phytochemicals to defend themselves from bacteria, fungi, viruses, and insects, as well as to heal tissues damaged by wind, sunburn, and other trauma. Because life processes are similar in all cells and organisms, you benefit from many of these phytochemicals when you eat plants. Of the thousands, perhaps millions, of phytochemicals in plants, only a small percentage have been analyzed for their functions in humans. Some are listed below.

- *Adenosine* is a blood thinner that guards against stroke and heart disease by preventing the formation of unnecessary blood clots. Clots may cause a heart attack or stroke. Adenosine is found in garlic, onions, and black mushrooms.
- *Ajoene* is another blood thinner also found in garlic.
- *Allicin*, which acts as an antibiotic and antifungal, also helps prevent the formation of cancer-causing nitrosamines in your stomach. Allicin is found in garlic and is responsible for its strong odor.
- *Bioflavonoids,* a group of 200-plus plant pigments, give citrus fruits their orange and yellow colors. Strong antioxidants that help the body ward off heart disease and cancer, bioflavonoids also strengthen the capillaries and reduce allergy-driven inflammation. Bioflavonoids are found in the skins and outer layers of fruits and vegetables, as well as in leafy vegetables, wine, tea, and coffee. You may have heard some of their individual names: catechin, hesperidin, quercetin, and rutin.

- *Capsaicin*, which gives chile peppers their hot flavor, helps us keep cool by reducing inflammation and pain. It can also ease cluster headaches, clear clogged breathing passages, protect cells from cancer-causing chemicals, reduce LDL cholesterol, and lower blood-fat (triglyceride) levels.
- *Catechins,* part of the bioflavonoid family, are in the news thanks to the increasing popularity of green tea, in which they are found. These bioflavonoids may help fight cancer, lower cholesterol and high blood pressure, combat bacteria, reduce high blood-glucose levels, and slow the aging process.
- *Coumarin,* like adenosine and ajoene, helps prevent heart disease and stroke by thinning the blood and aids the body in the battle against cancer. You'll find it in whole grains, fruits, and vegetables.
- *Ellagic acid* is a quiet soldier in the battle against cancer, helping to neutralize carcinogens before they damage healthy cells. Ellagic is a sweet phytochemical found in grapes, strawberries, cherries, and other fruits.
- *Genistein* is at least partially responsible for the anti-cancer properties attributed to soy and soy-based products such as tofu. It may help to fight the disease, especially cancers of the breast and uterus, by blocking the blood supply to tumors.
- *Glutathione* is an antioxidant found in tomatoes, watermelon, strawberries, and avocados. It fights free radicals, protects against cancer and heart disease, and slows the process of aging.
- *Indoles* are part of the "crucifer" family of vegetables' armament against cancer. The crucifers, which include broccoli, Brussels sprouts, cabbage, and cauliflower, have long been noted for their ability to help guard against colon cancer, breast cancer, and other forms of the disease.
- *Isoflavones* use their resemblance to estrogen to fight cancer. Certain breast and other tumors are nourished by estrogen, the female hormone. Isoflavones occupy estrogen receptors in tumor cells, which may help to prevent the real estrogen from entering. Isoflavones are found in peas, lentils, beans, and peanuts.

- *Lignans* fight cancer by deactivating the estrogen that seeks to feed tumors. They're also antioxidants that guard against damage by free radicals. Lignans are found in most plants.

- *Linolenic acid*, an essential fatty acid and powerful antioxidant, aids in the battle against heart disease, cancer, inflammation, and other ailments. It's found in fish, whole grains, soybeans, and most seeds.

- *Limonene* is found in the skins of citrus fruits. This little-noticed phytochemical may help inhibit or prevent certain cancerous growths.

- *Lycopene*, like capsaicin, is an antioxidant and a relative of beta-carotene, found in watermelon, tomatoes, red grapefruit, red peppers, and other red-colored fruits or vegetables. Lycopene may help guard against cancers of the prostate, colon, lung, bladder, and cervix. Lycopene is one of the antioxidants that keeps LDL in the bloodstream from being oxidized. One study found that people with the highest levels of lycopene were 48 percent less likely to have heart attacks. Cooking tomatoes makes the lycopene much easier for the body to assimilate. Therefore, tomato sauces or purees are better sources than fresh tomatoes.

- *Phenols* are a large group of antioxidant compounds that promote health in many ways, including helping to fight viruses, control excessive bleeding, and neutralize carcinogens. Garlic, soybeans, flaxseed, potatoes, citrus fruit, and green tea all contain phenols.

- *Phytates*, which are found in whole grains and soybeans, can help prevent the growth of certain tumors.

- *Phytoestrogens* protect against certain cancers by pretending to be estrogen. Like the isoflavones, they bind to special receptors on estrogen-dependent tumors, preventing the real thing from nourishing the unwanted growth. Eating beans and soy products, which contain phytoestrogens, has been linked to lower rates of breast cancer, as well as fewer deaths from cancer of the pancreas and prostate.

- *Protease inhibitors* help prevent the digestion of excessive amounts of protein. Protease inhibitors also assist in keeping cellular DNA from mutating and becoming cancerous. These cancer-fighting phytochemicals are found in soybeans, kidney beans, chickpeas, tofu, flax, and oats.

- *Quercetin*, an antioxidant found in red grapes, broccoli, onions, and shallots, helps to deactivate certain strong carcinogens and tumor promoters. When combined with vitamin C, it also can help fight off viruses.
- *Resveratrol* helps reduce the risk of heart disease and stroke by preventing the formation of unnecessary blood clots. It also may help to keep healthy cells from becoming cancerous, while inhibiting the spread of cancerous growths. Resveratrol is found in the skins of white and red grapes, as well as in red wine and red grape juice.
- *Sulfides* protect the heart and cardiovascular system by helping to keep blood pressure under control and thinning the blood. You'll find them in garlic, cabbage, broccoli, Brussels sprouts, and other vegetables.
- *Tannins* are acids found in tea that can help inhibit inflammation and guard against unnecessary blood clots.
- *Triterpenoids,* cancer-fighting phytochemicals found in licorice root and citrus fruits, can slow or prevent the growth of certain kinds of cancer by deactivating steroidal hormones.
- *Zeaxanthin* is a carotenoid found in dark green leafy vegetables, such as spinach. It may help to prevent some ailments, including macular degeneration, which can rob you of your sight.

All plants contain some substances that are helpful and some that are harmful to humans. Many phytochemicals are beneficial in small amounts and harmful in large amounts. Some are so toxic that eating just a small amount can make you sick or can even kill you, yet these phytochemicals may be used as medications. You cannot eat foxglove plants, for instance, but they are the source of digitalis, an important heart medication, which is given in tiny, carefully controlled doses.

Edible plants contain such small amounts of toxic phytochemicals that they are harmless to humans when eaten in reasonable amounts. But be careful not to overdo consumption of any one plant just because it is promoted as being healthful. Heart-health claims are made for oatmeal for its soluble fiber, flaxseeds for their omega-3 fatty acids, soybeans for their phytoestrogens, almonds for their monounsaturated fats, and so forth. If these claims lead you to include these and other plants in your diet, they are serving an educational purpose. If they cause you to consume LARGE amounts of a specific food, to limit your variety of other foods, or to take in too many calories, then these health claims can cause you to actually harm yourself.

I don't recommend selecting specific foods to get specific phytochemicals, or taking supplements containing phytochemicals extracted from plants. Once you realize the wide variety of phytochemicals that exist, their benefits, and all that we DON'T know about how they function and interact, I think you will agree that the best course is to eat as many different plants as possible. That way your body can select what it needs at any given time without being overloaded with any one substance that may have negative effects in large amounts. When you hear that a new phytochemical has been identified, don't buy pills or eat huge amounts of fruits or vegetables that contains the new substance. Just continue to eat a variety of fruits, vegetables, whole grains, beans, and other seeds, and you'll benefit from ALL of the phytochemicals.

TOO MUCH OF A GOOD THING?

Soybeans contain genistein, a weak plant estrogen that may help to prevent breast cancer. They contain omega-3 fatty acids, which help to prevent heart attacks, and fiber, which helps to prevent diabetes. Because these benefits have been demonstrated by science, soybean producers are allowed to print health claims on their labels.

But soybeans also contain trypsin inhibitors that block protein consumption and hemagglutinin, which causes clots to form. So large amounts of soybeans could make clots that can damage your heart or lungs. Trypsin inhibitors can block protein use and therefore make your pancreas

Vitamins for Heart Health

Vitamins are chemical compounds that the human body needs to grow and function normally. Of the thirteen vitamins humans need, eleven are abundant in plants. Your body gets most of its vitamin D from sunshine. (It's also found in milk, eggs, and fish.) Vitamin B-12 is found only in animals, but it is often added to plant-based foods, such as cereals or soy milk.

Most of the vitamins humans need are made in plants, so you get plenty when you eat a variety of fruits, vegetables, whole grains, beans, and other seeds. The B vitamins, thiamin, riboflavin, niacin, pyridoxine, folate, cyanocobalamin, pantothenic acid, and biotin, are needed to convert carbohydrates into energy, in addition to hundreds of other functions. They are found in whole grains, beans, and many plants, as well as in animals that eat these plants.

Vitamins A, C, and E are called the antioxidant vitamins, because one of their important jobs is to prevent certain oxidizing chemical reactions that can be harmful to your body. The antioxidant vitamins help to prevent heart disease, because LDL cholesterol must be oxidized before it can form plaque in your arteries. Brightly colored fruits and vegetables are particularly good sources of the antioxidant vitamins A and C. Whole grains and other seeds provide vitamin E.

You can get all the vitamins you need from the food you eat. A daily multivitamin for extra insurance won't hurt you, but don't believe that taking a vitamin pill will correct an unhealthful diet. Megadoses of vitamins or high-priced supplements that make extravagant promises are usually a waste of money, and problems can occur if you take too much of some vitamins. If you are concerned about low levels of vitamin D, because of lack of sunshine, or the B vitamins, your doctor can check these with a simple blood test.

work too hard to overcome this effect. Soy also contains goitrogens, which block thyroid function. In small doses these goitrogens do not harm you, but large doses can slow your thyroid. Soybeans and many other plants also contain phytates, which could block the absorption of minerals.

Don't take this information as a warning to avoid foods made with soybeans. The message is that all edible plants have the potential for harm if you eat them in large amounts. The concern is even greater if you are dealing with plant extracts in pills; you have no idea what or how much of any substance you are consuming. A healthful diet contains a wide variety of foods in moderate quantities. Don't eat five, ten, or twenty servings a day of any single food, no matter what promoters or advertisers say.

Minerals for Heart Health

Most of the minerals we need are the same ones plants require for their own growth: carbon, hydrogen, oxygen, nitrogen, phosphorous, potassium, sulfur, calcium, magnesium, iron, boron, manganese, copper, zinc, molybdenum, and chlorine.

Plants don't store minerals just for our benefit—they use them for their own life cycles. If any of their sixteen essential elements are not available, the plant withers and dies. When you buy any fruit or vegetable, you know that the plant grew successfully and had all of the minerals it needed. If you eat a wide variety of foods from plants, you will get plenty of all these minerals.

The minerals we need that plants don't are sodium, iodine, fluoride, selenium, and cobalt. These may be in plants, but the plants don't die if they're not available. Most people get plenty of these minerals, because our diet is abundant in salt, our water is fluoridated, and our food is grown in many different locations. Plants grown far from the oceans lack iodine, and a person who ate only these plants would have goiter, but this condition is no longer seen in North America, because we use iodized salt and eat foods from all parts of the continent. Following the DASH Plus guidelines should give you all of the minerals you need. If you and your doctor think you need extra calcium, see "Calcium Supplements" on the following page.

Calcium Supplements

You need calcium, but don't believe claims that it will cure heart disease, osteoporosis, or anything else. Lack of calcium can cause osteoporosis, but taking extra calcium does not treat it. If you're not confident that you are getting enough calcium in your diet, you can use fortified foods such as calcium-added orange juice, soy milk, or breakfast cereals, or you can take generic calcium carbonate pills. You don't need expensive chelated calcium pills, so-called "coral calcium," or supplements that combine magnesium with calcium. Magnesium is not necessary for calcium absorption. Coral calcium is just ordinary limestone, which offers no advantage over generic calcium carbonate or antacid tablets. Since calcium uses up vitamin D, people who take calcium supplements or antacids should also take vitamin D supplements.

DASH Plus Fitness—Week 7: Pick Up the Pace

Competitive athletes know that the only way that they can become stronger and faster is to increase the intensity of their workouts and exercise their muscles against greater resistance. Runners have to run very fast in practice and weight lifters have to lift very heavy weights. Use these same principles to improve your own exercise program.

You will become more fit by running a few miles quickly once or twice a week than by running many miles slowly. However, every time that you exercise intensely, your muscles are damaged, and it takes at least 48 hours for them to heal. That's why competitive athletes exercise intensely one to three times a week, and exercise at a more casual pace or take days off the rest of the time. If you want to become more fit, you need to do the same. On one day, you have to tax your muscles by exercising more intensely or by lifting heavier weights. The next day your muscles feel sore because they are actually damaged, so you have to exercise lightly or take the day off. And you continue to exercise lightly until your muscles do not feel sore. Then you exercise intensely again.

Be Realistic

Nobody can exercise vigorously in the same sport every day. If you think that you can, expect to get injured. Even top athletes use a program of hard days, easy days, and days off. But the hard-easy principle applies to your skeletal muscles, not to your heart. Athletes who are in very good shape can exercise hard on consecutive days as long as they do not use the same set of skeletal muscles—as top triathletes know. For everyone else, it's much better to exercise vigorously one day and then go easy or take off the next day than to just lollygag every day.

TRAINING IS SPECIFIC

Competitive athletes train in a single sport twelve months a year. If you have a favorite activity, concentrate on developing your muscles and endurance for that sport, because training is specific. The best way to become strong for cycling is to ride very fast, and ride up hills to work against resistance with exactly the same motions you use to pedal on level ground. Lifting weights with your legs does not make you as strong for cycling as pedaling intensely, because the muscle movements you make on a weight machine are different from those used to push the pedals. The harder you push on the pedals, the stronger you become for cycling. Competitive cyclists should ride very fast in short bursts, called intervals, once or twice a week.

Because my favorite sport is cycling, that's what I do all the time. Diana and I have a tandem bicycle, and we ride very hard one or two days a week. Then we take easy days or days off until we recover. If it's raining, icy, or snowing, we ride inside on a stationary bicycle. We go on cycling weekends and all our friends are riders, so our social life centers around cycling. We love group rides where we can go head-to-head with other riders to see who has improved and who is slacking off. I also do a daily weight-training routine of four to six upper body exercises that takes five to ten minutes. If you have a favorite sport, that's the kind of program I recommend for you. You're more likely to exercise for the rest of your life if your sport is fun for you, not something you do just because you know it's good for you. Here's our program, which would work for any sport:

Saturday: Short, fast time trial
Sunday: Long and hard
Monday: Day off
Tuesday: Easy recovery day
Wednesday: Hills
Thursday: Easy
Friday: Easy

CROSS-TRAINING

If you want to become very good in your favorite sport, I recommend doing only that activity plus a weight training program that complements it. However, some people prefer variety and have a wide range of outdoor interests. If this describes you, choose two or more different sports, preferably one that targets the lower body, such as running, and one that works the upper body, such as rowing. Work out vigorously in each sport once a week, then work out lightly the rest of the time, taking off one or two days a week. Here's an example:

Monday: Aerobic dancing (lower body), moderate pace
Tuesday: Rowing (upper body), vigorous pace
Wednesday: Aerobic dancing (lower body), moderate pace

Thursday: Rowing (upper body), moderate pace
Friday: Aerobic dancing (lower body), vigorous pace
Saturday: Day off
Sunday: Day off

With this program, you stress the major muscle groups to the maximum only once a week—those of the upper body on Tuesday and those of the lower body on Friday. You never work the same muscle group two days in a row. And you're taking a complete rest for two days to give your body a chance to recover.

INTERVAL TRAINING FOR EVERYONE

Top athletes in all sports use a technique called interval training, and you can apply it to your program at any level of fitness. When you start a new exercise program, exercise for thirty seconds, then stop for 30 to 60 seconds or longer if you need it. Alternate exercising and resting until you feel tired or your muscles feel heavy. Then stop for the day.

> ➤ A NOTE FROM DR. GABE

Interval training can be used for every sport at every level of fitness. It's used by almost all competitive athletes.

The stronger you get in your sport, the more intense your interval workouts can become. You work at your maximum capacity for 30 to 60 seconds, then take 60 to 90 seconds to recover, then exercise vigorously for another 30 to 60 seconds. More than forty years ago, the Swedish physiologist Per Olof Astrand showed that you can increase your exercise load just by alternating short bursts of exercise with rest periods. Do this vigorous interval workout once a week until you get tired. At first you

One Fit, One Not So Fit? Try a Tandem Bicycle

Many couples don't exercise together because one partner is more fit than the other. Riding a tandem bicycle is a great equalizer.

The amount of work you do on a bicycle depends on how hard you push on the pedals. Pushing twice as hard on the pedals does twice the work, so a world-class bicycle racer can ride with a novice and still get a good workout. Even a beginner will be able to keep up with the spinning pedals, no matter how fast they go. The less-fit partner just applies little or no pressure, so he or she will not get tired. No matter how hard one partner tries to outcycle the other, they will always be together.

You can go faster together than the more-fit person can go alone. The more experienced rider sits in the front seat. If both people are equally good riders, the taller one usually sits in front. The person who sits in the back copies the motions of the person in the front. At first it may seem strange not to have any control over steering, shifting, or braking, but you have the big advantage of being able to exercise only as hard as you like while enjoying the scenery.

may be able to do only two or three intervals, but as your muscles get stronger, you build up the number of intervals. Remember, go easy the next day or take a day off if you feel any discomfort.

DASH Plus Food—Week 7: Finding Thyme

Everyone is busy! Once you make a commitment to eating healthfully, start collecting strategies that make preparing your own food fit into your schedule. Sometimes convenience costs more, but if you work long hours it can be worth it. Check out the stores and restaurants near you, and decide what works for your personal situation. Use your notebook to jot down ideas. Here are a few of my favorite tips for DASH Plus eating on hectic days.

1. Find a whole-grain cereal that tastes good dry, and eat it for breakfast on the run or for snacks. See the list of recommended cereals on page 179.

2. Make your own fast food. Once a week, cook a huge pot of chili, soup, or one of my vegetable or seafood casseroles. Freeze the leftovers in individual serving containers for quick suppers or lunches.

3. Cook a pound of whole grains, and freeze the leftovers in ½- to 1-cup portions in resealable plastic bags. These can be reheated in the microwave in seconds.

4. Stock up on soup cups that have dried beans or lentils as their main ingredient. Find flavors you like and use them for lunch at the office or on the run—anywhere you can get hot water. Mix the soup with one of the plastic bags of whole grains for a hearty main dish.

5. Find a few raw veggies that you like and eat them as you would fruit. Try red bell peppers, green beans, and cauliflower.

6. Romaine hearts, packed in plastic bags, can be used as is for quick salad preparation. Just tear or slice the lettuce into bite-size pieces. It's good even without dressing.

7. Most Asian restaurants offer carry-out service. This is a good standby for lazy days. Vietnamese restaurants often have wonderful, oil-free salads that keep for two to three days. Comb through the menu for soups, vegetables, seafood dishes, and steamed entrées. Ask them to go easy on the oil. Serve them atop those stored whole grains from your freezer.

8. Large grocery stores and specialty food stores often have salad bars and prepared-food sections. You need to be careful about your choices, but if you are strong willed, and not too hungry when you

shop, you can usually find plenty of vegetables, fruits, and possibly some seafood entrées among the offerings.

9. Take advantage of precut vegetables and fruits in your supermarket's produce department and bags of mixed vegetables in the frozen-food section. The time you save in the kitchen can make up for the added cost.

> **A NOTE FROM DR. GABE**

MUNCHY-CRUNCHY SNACKS: The best DASH Plus snacks are small portions of the good food choices you make for all your meals. If you like munchy-crunchy snacks, try:

- Air-popped popcorn (season with your favorite spice blend, not butter)
- Dry cereal, straight from the box
- Raw vegetables and salsa or bean dip
- Peanut butter on apple slices, celery, or carrots

Convenient energy sources while exercising include trail mixes, dried fruits, or nuts.

HERBS, SPICES, AND SEASONINGS

Many of the phytochemicals that have healthy heart benefits (see pages 134–135) are found in herbs and spices. The plants that have the most pungent flavors and scents are often the most concentrated sources of phytochemicals. You help your heart and your taste buds when you use a wide variety of edible herbs and spices that are available in any supermarket. This week's recipes encourage you to try some spicy foods and combinations that may be new to you.

➤ A NOTE FROM DR. GABE

Create a DASH Plus clipping file—in a drawer or on your
computer—for recipe ideas, interesting health or food articles,
and useful Web sites.

Many different cultures base their diets on the foods in the DASH
Plus program, so you will find a wide array of ethnic recipes that fit my
guidelines. Healthful eating is more fun if you sample all of these fasci-
nating cuisines, in restaurants and in your own home. If the spices and
seasoning combinations are new to you, try them a few times before you
make your final judgment. Some tastes take a while to acquire.

Heat in most recipes and spice mixes comes from ground hot peppers,
but you can always adjust the level of spiciness to your taste. Start with a
tiny bit and then add more, if you wish. Put a bottle of hot pepper sauce
on the table so others in your family can get the degree of heat they like.

Spice Blends

Spice blends such as curry powder, chili powder, and Cajun spice are a great
shortcut for the busy cook who wants maximum taste with minimum effort.
Use them to add infinite variety to your combinations of whole grains, beans,
fruits, and vegetables. Look for mild curry or chili powders and add the degree
of heat you want with a little cayenne pepper or hot sauce, such as Tabasco.
If you don't like one spice blend, try another brand; each manufacturer has its
own formula, and most supermarkets carry several brands. Or you can make
your own using my recipes at www.healthyheartmiracle.com.

Featured Recipes • Week 7
Ethnic and Spicy Dishes

Menu Plan • Week 7   See Weekly Menu Plans

WEEK 8

Your Personal DASH Plus Lifestyle Plan

The last week of the 8-Week Plan can be the beginning of a life-long DASH Plus lifestyle for a healthy heart. Turn the changes you've made in the past seven weeks into permanent habits, and you will reap all the benefits of good nutrition and exercise. At the end of the week you'll fill in the 8th Week column of your Before and After Progress Worksheet, so call your doctor's office or lab to schedule an appointment to get your blood values checked.

Even before you know your latest test results, I'll bet that you are delighted with the way you feel and what you see in the mirror. Eating the DASH Plus way gives you more energy, and you probably are sleeping better and feel full of vigor because of your new exercise program. Knowing that you have taken control of your cholesterol, blood pressure, and blood sugar is tremendously satisfying.

This week is devoted to personalizing all of my recommendations to fit your specific situation. Then you'll map out an action plan that will remind you where you should concentrate your attention, where and how often you can "cheat," and which concerns don't apply to you. But before we get started, lift up your arm, bend your elbow and give yourself a resounding pat on the back. You've earned it!

Your Heart-Health Priorities

The basics of a heart-healthy lifestyle are the same for everyone: eat lots of plants, and get plenty of vigorous exercise. These essentials apply to everyone from toddlers to centenarians. What else you do—or don't do—depends on your personal health and your family history. Which of these statements did you pick to describe yourself at the beginning of the 8-Week Plan?

 I'm standing on the edge of a cliff. ☐

If you have had a heart attack or stroke, or have diabetes that is out of control, or have had bypass surgery or other procedures to unblock clogged arteries, your life is in jeopardy. You need to make the heart-health lifestyle changes your TOP PRIORITY. If you want to see your grandchildren grow up and want to dance at their weddings, don't slack off until ALL OF YOUR TESTS ARE NORMAL, your weight is where it belongs, and you can see your muscles. If you are highly motivated and work carefully with your doctor, you may be able to get off all or most of your medications. Your doctor will brag about you as a star patient.

STILL SMOKING? MORE THAN 100 POUNDS OVERWEIGHT? I'd put you in the Standing on the Edge of a Cliff group, even if you have no other heart-health issues. Smokers, read page 155; if you're severely obese, see page 159.

 I have one or more warning signs, but no heart-health crises yet. ☐

You're in this group if any of your tests from Week 1 were high, you are a diabetic who is well controlled, you are taking blood pressure or cholesterol-lowering medication, or your doctor has identified any other risk factors. Count yourself in this group if you have excess weight stored around your belly or have Polycystic Ovary Syndrome (see page 45). You can improve the quality of your life by continuing with the DASH Plus lifestyle plan. I work with my patients to get them off all medications or, at the very least, reduce their medication to the absolute minimum, and I think you should have the same goal for yourself. But you need to be motivated. Focus your efforts on the intensity of your exercise program and follow the DASH Plus guidelines as closely as you can. If you have more weight to lose, try to make steady progress. You will soon find out how much you can "cheat" without back-sliding. See "The 19 Meals for Dr. Gabe Rule" on page 165.

I'm basically healthy and want to stay that way.

Concentrate on developing and maintaining a lifetime sport that you truly love and look forward to doing as often as possible. The more active you are, the more food you can eat without heart-health consequences. Lifetime weight control and muscle strength depend more on physical activity than on diet; active people can eat pretty much whatever they want as long as they include plenty of the foods from the DASH Plus guidelines.

If you're basically healthy but are working to help a loved one who is in the "edge of a cliff" or "warning signs" category, your personal plan will focus on strategies to make changes in that person's personal lifestyle, with or without his or her awareness and participation. Use the Personal Roadmap for a Loved One (page 174).

REDUCING STRESS

You may be surprised that I've waited until the last week of the 8-Week Plan to talk about stress, considering that so many people believe it's a leading cause of heart attacks. I can measure your fitness and your nutritional status objectively, and I can tell you about hundreds of scientific studies on the effects of diet and exercise. But stress is subjective. What one person considers stressful may be a motivating source of success to another. A situation that causes you great distress may be just a minor annoyance for someone else. We don't have any reliable way to measure stress, and we don't even have a consensus of what constitutes stress or of what factors eliminate it.

Several studies associate stress with increased risk for heart attacks, and one study from Duke University showed that stress-reduction techniques reduce second heart attacks. If you and your doctor think that you may benefit from stress-management techniques, by all means use them, but ADD them to your food and fitness efforts. Stress-management programs may include meditation, education about heart disease and stress, training in stress-reduction skills, anger management, group support, yoga or Tai Chi classes, and/or tranquilizing medications.

It's my personal belief that telling patients their health problems are caused by stress is an example of blaming the victim. There's no doubt that your physical health and your overall happiness are intimately connected. If YOU are dissatisfied with your work or your personal relationships, if you do not have fulfilling interests and a sense of purpose, your health may suffer. But if I AS YOUR DOCTOR tell you your problem is caused by stress, it's often because I can't find any other physical explanation and don't want to admit that I don't know. I KNOW you can improve your heart health with diet and exercise, that's why I suggest focusing on these tangible changes. Good food choices and vigorous exercise are two of the best ways we have to combat stress, improve your mood, help you sleep more soundly, and feel better about yourself. Seeking counseling and making changes in your relationships, job, or environment may reduce your stress and thus help you to prevent heart attacks or strokes, but make these changes in conjunction with the DASH Plus guidelines and treatment plan.

Depression and panic attacks are treatable medical conditions that can increase your risk for heart attacks. If you suffer from either of these, please check with your doctor.

Depression, Fat, and Heart Attacks

A study from Washington University in St. Louis shows that people who are depressed have higher blood levels of C-Reactive Protein and interleukin-6, two measures of inflammation that predict an increased risk for heart attacks (explained in Week 6). The depressed subjects did not have higher rates of known causes of inflammation, such as cigarette smoking or infection, but they were significantly fatter than the control subjects. The authors believe that the excess fat, and not the depression, caused the high blood levels of inflammatory markers, and that being overweight is a more significant risk for a heart attack than being just depressed. They did not offer an opinion on possible links between being depressed and being overweight.

Depression and Omega-3s

Postpartum depression is common, and pregnancy requires large amounts of omega-3 fatty acids. Women with the lowest blood levels of omega-3s are the ones most likely to suffer postpartum depression. Several studies have shown that depressed people often have low blood levels of omega-3s. If these studies can be supported, some cases of depression may be prevented and treated by eating deepwater fish, whole grains, beans, nuts, and other seeds.

USING DASH PLUS FOR LONG-TERM WEIGHT LOSS AND WEIGHT CONTROL

Almost everyone who follows the DASH Plus guidelines will lose weight if he or she is overweight. Even though the DASH Diet was not designed specifically for weight loss, most people take in significantly fewer calories when they eat this way compared to their old eating patterns. The changes I made when I modified the DASH guidelines to create the DASH Plus plan favor additional weight loss: whole grains instead of refined grain products, fewer saturated fats, and, of course, your exercise program.

If You're Still Smoking

I didn't suggest that you quit smoking at the beginning of the 8-Week Plan because I knew it would make you cranky and you'd find it hard to focus on anything else. Now that you've spent the last several weeks learning new ways to eat and exercise, why not take the REALLY BIG step that will improve your health more than anything else you do? Aside from the lung cancer risk, smoking doubles your chances of having a heart attack or stroke. Within just a couple of years after you quit, your heart attack risk is no greater than that of a person who has never smoked.

Anyone who still smokes in the twenty-first century knows all of the consequences and knows that quitting is tough. But other people succeed, and so can you. Your doctor may be able to give you some specific suggestions and direct you to local resources, but whatever method you choose, expect the first few weeks to be the worst. Prepare your family and your co-workers and ask for their support. At www.healthyheartmiracle.com you'll find links to national organizations that can help. Then do it!

Any eating plan that is designed to make you take in fewer calories than you burn will cause you to lose weight. The beauty of the DASH Plus guidelines is that not only do you lose weight, you get all of the nutrients from your food that your body needs. This means you can eat this way permanently. Use "The 19 Meals for Dr. Gabe Rule" (page 165) to keep yourself motivated.

No matter what authors of popular diets may tell you, the basic equation for weight loss is CALORIES IN < CALORIES BURNED. You can reduce your intake of calories, increase the number you burn with more vigorous exercise, or both. The DASH Plus guidelines emphasize the importance of exercise because it's virtually impossible to take off weight and keep it off for life just by restricting food.

You need to eat a certain amount of varied foods to provide the nutrients your body needs. If you eat less than that you develop deficiencies, and your body goes into starvation mode, working to conserve calories by slowing down your metabolism. That's why drastic low-calorie diets are not healthful and don't work. With DASH Plus you never feel hungry and you get all the nutrients you need. The more active you are, the more food you can eat and still lose weight.

WHAT IF I'M NOT LOSING WEIGHT?

When you first start an exercise program, the weight-loss benefits probably will not be immediately obvious. That's because your muscles are still weak, you don't have much endurance, and you're not burning many calories, even though you're exerting what seems like a tremendous amount of effort. Don't let this discourage you. Within weeks, the exercise routine that had you huffing and puffing will seem too easy. Then you'll know it's time to pick up the pace. Every few weeks or months the same thing will happen: What once was hard becomes easy, and you'll need to add more speed or resistance to your routine. And all the while your heart muscle is getting stronger, your lung capacity is improving, and you are burning more calories.

While you are working up to the point where you can exercise vigorously enough to lose a significant amount of weight, you can adjust the number of DASH Plus servings to reduce your total calorie intake, but you don't need to count calories, or grams of carbohydrates, fat, or protein. The numbers and sizes of servings are based on the intake of an average-size person, so if you are small, try cutting back on the number of servings of any of the foods except vegetables. But for long-term weight control, I can't overemphasize the importance of regular, vigorous activity.

FIND A SPORT YOU TRULY LOVE

Whether or not weight control is one of your goals, your long-range plans should include a sport or recreational activity that you will still be able to enjoy when you're eighty, ninety, and beyond. If you began your DASH Plus Fitness program with walking, you may want to proceed to brisker, longer walks, and perhaps even to racewalking. Stick with it into your golden years. The Senior Olympics await you!

However, the first sport you pick may not be your lifetime sport. Branch out and try other activities until you find one that suits you. Since you chose an activity to start the 8-Week Plan, you've built up your endurance, skeletal muscle strength, and heart strength. That means starting another sport will be easier for you, because your overall level of fitness is higher. Keep your eyes open for activities you haven't tried yet, or return to sports you may have learned as a child. For example, if you knew how to swim or ride a bike, those skills are still there, lodged in your brain, even if you haven't used them in years. You would be rusty at first, but a few practice sessions will get you going again. But do keep in mind that anytime you start a new sport you need to begin gradually, no matter how fit you are. Every sport uses different muscles, and you can get injured easily if you don't strengthen the muscles your new activity requires.

In Week 3, I made some suggestions for making any exercise program more fun, but now I want to discuss passion. Some people stay married to their first love for seventy-five years, while others take two, three, or more tries to find the perfect lifetime partner. It's the same with exercise. If you think it's too late for you to find a sport you truly love, not one you do just because you know it's good for you, read about Diana's trike on page 163. Then keep looking for a sport that makes you feel the same way.

DIET GIMMICKS

Before you waste your money and your time on the latest diet gimmick, use the old rule, "If it sounds too good to be true, it probably is."

- There are no creams that will dissolve fat.
- Eating collagen before you sleep does not make your body burn fat.

- Fat absorbers (chitin products) do bind to small amounts of fat, but they cost about $35 to block the fat in one Big Mac.
- If carbohydrate blockers actually worked, you would have explosive diarrhea, cramping, and gas from the undigested carbs being attacked by bacteria in your colon.
- Pills or anything that promises to get rid of cellulite are useless. Cellulite doesn't exist, it's just ordinary fat.
- Products that remove water (diuretics) or empty your colon (laxatives or colon cleansers) can cause you to drop several pounds in a day or two, but this is temporary and does not remove any fat. You do not

Minority Report: Gain Muscle, Not Fat

So many people are overweight that anyone who wants to gain weight gets little sympathy. If you think you're too thin and want to gain weight, don't just sit on the couch and stuff yourself with food. Weight gain should always be in the form of muscle, not fat. To build muscle, start a weight-bearing exercise program (see page 120). As you build muscle, your appetite will respond to meet your needs. It takes only 15 extra grams of protein a day to build a pound of muscle a week—so you really won't need to eat a lot more.

It's never too late to start a weight-training program. Underweight older people look and feel frail because they have lost most of their muscle mass, not because of lack of fat. If you are inactive, you lose muscle mass to the point where you are unable to carry out daily activities, such as climbing stairs or getting up out of a chair, because your muscles are not strong enough to move the weight of your own body. Don't try to add fat to a weak body. Overweight older people often have the double burden of weak muscles *AND* twenty, forty, or more extra pounds to lug around every day. Muscles are vital whether you are thin or heavy because they are your immune system's reservoir.

need to "cleanse" or "remove toxic waste products" to lose weight, or for any other reason. Prolonged use of diuretics or laxatives can be dangerous.

- Most products that claim to "rev up your metabolism" or "burn fat" contain stimulants. Many plants contain stimulants, and you will get the same effect from drinking large amounts of coffee or tea as you will from "natural" or herbal weight loss products. Stimulants cause you to burn more calories, and you will lose weight at first, but you need to take more of them as the days go by, and they can cause unpleasant, even dangerous side effects.

IF YOU'RE MORE THAN 100 POUNDS OVERWEIGHT

We all love dramatic before-and-after stories of people who have lost huge amounts of weight, but the truth is that people who are more than 100 pounds overweight have little chance of losing and keeping weight off just with diet and exercise. They are different from other people, and they are at high risk for many diseases and premature death. While nobody really knows why these people are different, two hormones, ghrelin and leptin, are suspect. The only consistently effective treatment available today for morbid obesity is stomach bypass surgery, and it has risks of its own.

Your stomach releases a hormone called ghrelin that makes you hungry. Bypass surgery prevents food from entering your stomach, which stops the production of ghrelin and makes you feel less hungry. The other hormone, leptin, is produced by fat cells when they fill with fat. It acts on your brain to make you feel full. Scientists think that some cases of morbid obesity may be caused by an inability of the brain to respond to leptin. Drug companies are racing to solve the riddle of obesity, because a successful drug will be worth billions of dollars.

Anyone who tells morbidly obese people that they are too fat because they eat too much or exercise too little is callous and unrealistic. While we await a breakthrough, the only effective treatment medical science has to offer is stomach bypass surgery. Talk to your doctor to see if you are a candidate.

THREE WEEKS TO CHANGE A HABIT

Behavior researchers tell us that it takes only three weeks to change a habit. If that's true, think what you've accomplished in eight weeks of work on your eating and exercise routines! If you like the results, keep these new habits and build on them for the rest of your life. Use the Personal Roadmap to map out what you've already accomplished, what needs monitoring, and what needs your long-term attention.

DASH Plus Fitness—Week 8: The Fountain of Youth

In 1490, Ponce de Leon set out to find the fountain of youth. He didn't succeed, and more than 500 years later, the only mechanism to delay the signs of aging is exercise. There are no data to show that antioxidants, vitamins, or anything else prolongs life. All tests that are used to measure aging actually measure physical fitness. A fit 70-year-old will score "younger" on aging tests than an out-of-shape 20-year-old.

Scientists measure aging with a test called VO_2max, which gauges your maximal ability to take in and use oxygen. Many studies show that exercise maintains fitness. People who do not exercise lose 15 percent of their fitness per decade, those who exercise at low intensity lose 9 percent, while those who exercise intensely lose barely any fitness.

A study from India showed that former athletes who continued to exercise all their lives were far less likely to suffer heart attacks than former athletes who did not continue to exercise. Compared to sedentary former athletes, the older active athletes weighed less and had less body fat. They also had lower total cholesterol, bad LDL cholesterol, and triglyceride levels, as well as a better ratio of total cholesterol to HDL cholesterol—all signs of decreased risk for heart attacks. Surprisingly, the sedentary former athletes had higher cholesterol and triglyceride levels than sedentary older nonathletes. It takes a lot of muscle to be a good athlete. Insulin, insulin-like growth factors, and growth hormones give people large muscles and bones to make them stronger. However, these same hormones also cause the body to store fat (see the explanation of Syndrome X on page 44). Former athletes who stop exercising are more likely to be fat and have higher cholesterol because of these same hormones. So if you were a great athlete when you were younger, it's doubly important for you to keep exercising as you age.

EXERCISE FOR LIFETIME WEIGHT CONTROL

You know that you burn more calories when you're active than when you're sitting on the couch, but you may not realize that exercising also causes you to burn more calories during the rest of the day. Every time you exercise, your body temperature rises and stays elevated for up to 18 hours. During those hours, your body has a revved-up metabolism, so you burn calories at a higher rate.

Only vigorous exercise that increases body temperature and makes you sweat will increase your metabolism enough to continue burning more calories after you finish. Swimming, which is an excellent activity for strengthening your heart and for overall fitness, is not the best exercise for weight loss. Water conducts heat away from your body so your temperature doesn't rise, meaning you don't get the same metabolism-boosting effect that you get from exercising on land.

Exercise also helps you lose weight and keep it off because it increases the amount of muscle tissue, and muscles burn more calories than fat. However, muscles are heavier than fat, so if you exercise a lot, don't be surprised if your scales don't show as much of a loss as you expect.

Instead of the scale, use your tape measure and your eyes to monitor your progress.

INTENSITY FOR WEIGHT LOSS

Some people recommend that you exercise at a slow rate because you burn a greater percentage of fat than when you exercise intensely. This doesn't make sense because when you exercise at a low level of intensity, you burn fewer calories during and after exercise, so the total number of calories you burn in a 24-hour period is far less. Burning fewer calories causes you to lose less weight.

WALK OR RUN FOR WEIGHT LOSS?

Do you burn the same number of calories if you run or walk the same distance? It depends on how fast you walk. When you run, you burn about 100 calories per mile, no matter how fast you go. You keep the same running form at any speed. When you walk slowly, at three miles an hour, you burn about 65 calories per mile. When you walk fast, at five miles an hour, you burn about 128 calories per mile. The faster you walk, with the exaggerated side-to-side motion, the more energy you use. Fast walking can be even more vigorous than running, and you are less likely to be injured.

USE IT OR LOSE IT

All of the benefits you gain from exercise are lost soon after you stop. Muscles enlarged by lifting heavy weights return to their previous size within a few weeks after you stop lifting, and people who do aerobic exercise have slow heart rates and greater endurance for only a short time after they stop their program. But once you're in good shape, you can be fit into old age just by continuing your exercise program, working muscles

Diana's Fitness Story: My Trike

I was always the last child picked for teams in elementary school. I hated gym in high school, and I did nothing athletic in college. As an adult I swam a little and took some aerobic dance classes, but my idea of vigorous activity was chasing after my children. Starting at age 50, under my husband's patient guidance, it took me several years to get comfortable enough on our tandem bicycle so that I could get a good workout. I got noticeably stronger and started to be more than just a dead weight on the bicycle. Riding in tandem is wonderful because we travel through beautiful countryside, and I look forward to all our trips. Unfortunately, though, I can ride only when my husband is available.

So last year, at age 61, I got the idea of using a recumbent trike as a way to run one of our dogs that needed lots of exercise. It was so much fun that when I finished riding alongside the dog for five miles or so, I'd take him home and then keep on going. The beauty of a trike for someone like me is that there's no balance problem, no risk of falling, virtually no skill needed at all. You can move as fast or as slow as you like, and climbing hills is easy because you can shift into a very low gear. It's a serious machine, not a toy (mine is from Australia, where they're popular for racing). Kids of all ages think it's "cool." (See the photos at www.healthyheartmiracle.com.)

I take my trike through the neighborhood to the local trails, where I can go as far as I like. I've created my own program of long days, fast days, intervals, and recovery days. Because I don't have any sports injuries to hold me back, I ride more than my husband and I'm not tied to his schedule. The strength in my legs has doubled since I started on the trike and that's improved my tandem riding, too. But the big advantage is—it's so much fun! I arrange my days so I can ride as much as possible, and if the sun is shining all my other plans get cancelled; I'm out on my trike.

against resistance a few minutes a day. I hope the results you've seen in the last eight weeks convince you that it's worth the effort.

> ➤ **A NOTE FROM DR. GABE**
>
> Your body is a wonderful machine, designed to last 120 years or more.

DASH Plus Food—Week 8: How Much Can You Cheat?

When you use the DASH Plus guidelines to control diabetes, cholesterol, or high blood pressure, you need to be stricter than someone who just wants to stay healthy. But I don't expect ANYONE to be perfect. If you sustain your healthful habits most of the time, you can do whatever you like once in a while.

You've spent this week evaluating your goals and setting priorities for yourself, for both your exercise program and your long-term eating regimen. Review these goals often and stick to your plan. I think you'll quickly figure out just how often you can "slide" without getting off track. If you're in the "Edge of a Cliff" category, use "The 19 Meals for Dr. Gabe Rule" and limit your "cheats" to no more than one or two meals a week.

SUPPORT YOUR LOVED ONE

When one person in a household is in danger, and the spouse, children, and other family members are basically healthy, the needs of the person in trouble should dominate the family's food choices. The healthy members can cheat elsewhere. Keep the refrigerator and kitchen cabinets stocked with heart-healthy foods.

The 19 Meals for Dr. Gabe Rule

If you follow the DASH Plus guidelines faithfully for nineteen out of your twenty-one meals per week, you can eat out once or twice and have anything you want for the other two meals. Be reasonable, don't stuff yourself, but enjoy your food without guilt. If you haven't been able to change your eating habits in the past, you'll find that this simple rule makes a big difference.

- You can eat at friends' homes without asking them to cater to your special food needs.
- You can satisfy a craving for a favorite food.
- You can enjoy a lunchtime or evening at a restaurant with family or coworkers.
- Your holidays and celebrations can include your family's favorite foods.

Notice that I said eat OUT once or twice. When you order a bacon-lettuce-and-tomato sandwich at a deli, you eat two slices of bread and two slices of bacon. If you make it yourself at home, you need to buy a loaf of bread and a pound of bacon. Who's going to eat the rest? Keep your house temptation-free.

CELEBRATE! BUFFET-STYLE MEALS FOR FAMILY OR ENTERTAINING

In our house we have one-dish meals, two-dish meals, and buffet-style meals. The Mix and Match Salad is an example of a one-dish meal, in which all of the ingredients are tossed together. The two-dish meal, as I explained in Week 4, is usually a hot dish plus a salad, because no matter how many different kinds of cooked vegetables go into one of my vegetable stews or seafood casseroles, you should still eat some leafy greens.

The buffet-style meal usually comes after several days of accumulating leftovers, but it's also great for entertaining. For a buffet meal, serve several dishes—appetizers, soups, salads, main dishes, desserts—in no particular order. Just put them all on the table and let your family or your guests pick whatever appeals to them.

You may not think that the recipes in the 8-Week Plan would have much party appeal, but for this week's menus I've included recipes that have proven to be favorites for casual entertaining or even as part of a festive holiday buffet. All of these recipes are easy to double or triple if you're expecting a crowd.

> ➤ **A NOTE FROM DR. GABE**
>
> DASH Plus is not a diet! It's a way of moving, eating, and living.

Featured Recipes—Week 8
Party Buffet

Smoked Salmon Salad	Page 206
Wild Rice Fruit Salad	Page 209
Maryland Crab Soup	Page 216
Sweet Potato Bisque	Page 220
Chafing Dish Chili	Page 225
Paprika Casserole	Page 230
Penang Shrimp Curry	Page 231
Fruity Pebbles	Page 239
Gingered Fruit Compote	Page 238
Fruit Kabobs	Page 238
Fresh Salsa	Page 245
Guacamole	Page 246
Easy Spicy Peanut Dip	Page 244

Menu Plan • Week 8   See Weekly Menu Plans

The Healthy Heart Miracle
Personal Roadmap

To download Personal Roadmap forms, go to www. healthyheartmiracle.com.

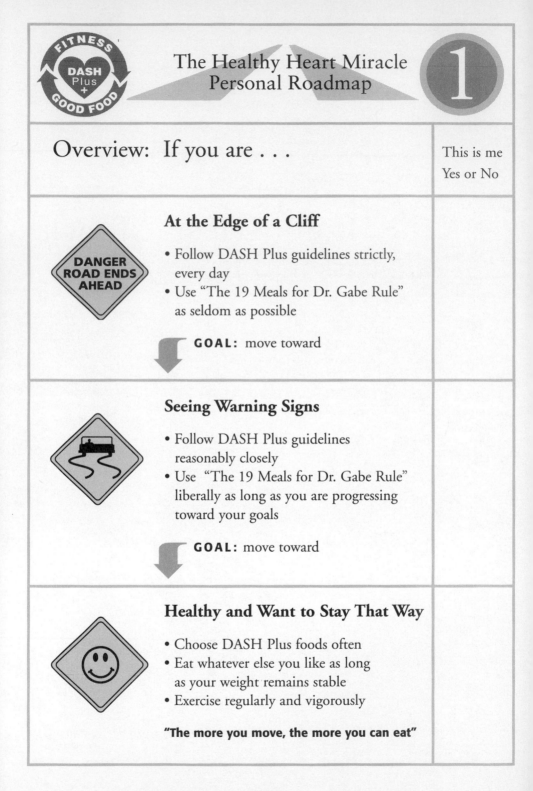

The Healthy Heart Miracle Personal Roadmap

1

Overview: If you are . . .	This is me Yes or No

At the Edge of a Cliff

DANGER ROAD ENDS AHEAD

- Follow DASH Plus guidelines strictly, every day
- Use "The 19 Meals for Dr. Gabe Rule" as seldom as possible

GOAL: move toward

Seeing Warning Signs

- Follow DASH Plus guidelines reasonably closely
- Use "The 19 Meals for Dr. Gabe Rule" liberally as long as you are progressing toward your goals

GOAL: move toward

Healthy and Want to Stay That Way

- Choose DASH Plus foods often
- Eat whatever else you like as long as your weight remains stable
- Exercise regularly and vigorously

"The more you move, the more you can eat"

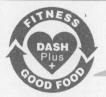

The Healthy Heart Miracle
Personal Roadmap

2

FITNESS STRATEGIES—BEGINNER

NOTE: BE SURE TO CHECK WITH YOUR DOCTOR OR HEALTHCARE PROVIDER BEFORE BEGINNING AN EXERCISE PROGRAM.

	NEED TO DO	ALREADY DONE	DOES NOT APPLY TO ME
Measure myself—BMI, Waist/Hip Ratio, and Inch of Pinch Test *(see Week 1)*			
Assess my fitness level *(see Week 1)*			
Choose at least one activity or sport from list *(see Week 2)*			
Work up to 30 minutes sustained activity in my chosen sport *(see Week 2)*			
Keep a daily journal to track my progress (time, intensity, days off, any injuries, etc.) *(see Worksheet)*			
Warm up and cool down each time I work out *(see Week 5)*			
Stretch after muscles are warmed up *(see Week 5)*			
Begin or continue weight-training program *(see Week 6)*			
Try a new sport or activity *(see Weeks 2 and 8)*			
Join a club, class, or group activity for exercise			
Buy the piece of exercise equipment I have selected and tried *(see Worksheet)*			
Make my program more fun			
Find and involve AT LEAST ONE DASH Plus partner—spouse, other family member, friend— in my fitness program, food program, or both			

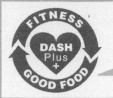

The Healthy Heart Miracle
Personal Roadmap

3

FITNESS STRATEGIES—EXPERIENCED EXERCISERS

NOTE: BE SURE TO CHECK WITH YOUR DOCTOR OR HEALTHCARE PROVIDER BEFORE BEGINNING AN EXERCISE PROGRAM.

	NEED TO DO	ALREADY DONE	DOES NOT APPLY TO ME
Keep a daily journal to track my progress (time, intensity, days off, any injuries, etc.) *(see Week 2)*			
Maintain my current program with hard and easy days *(see Week 2)*			
Increase number of session/days per week? *(see Week 3)*			
Increase distance? *(see Week 3)*			
Start interval training program *(see Week 7)*			
Add another sport or change sports based on questionnaire *(see Worksheet)*			
Start or increase a weight-training program *(see Week 6)*			
Join a new club, group, or class related to my existing program or a new sport *(see Week 3)*			
Make my program more fun *(see Week 3)*			
Train for/begin/increase program for races, games, competition			
Find and involve at least one DASH Plus partner			

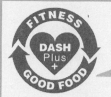

The Healthy Heart Miracle
Personal Roadmap

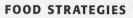

4

FOOD STRATEGIES

	NEED TO DO	ALREADY DONE	DOES NOT APPLY TO ME
Clean out kitchen/keep it temptation free! *(see Week 1)*			
Stock cupboards and freezer with DASH Plus foods *(see Worksheet)*			
Try new DASH Plus recipes each week			
Buy a countertop steamer to make preparing whole grains and vegetables easier *(see Week 4)*			
Find and eat at DASH Plus–friendly restaurants *(see Week 6)*			
Patronize food stores and restaurants that offer healthful choices (vote with your dollars) *(see Week 6)*			
Share recipe success with others (have a party, trade, and share leftovers)			
Find and involve AT LEAST ONE DASH Plus partner —spouse, other family member, friend—in my Fitness program, Food program or BOTH			

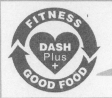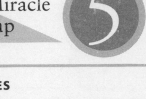

The Healthy Heart Miracle
Personal Roadmap

5

SPECIFIC FOOD STRATEGIES

	HIGH BLOOD PRES- SURE	HIGH LDL	LOW LDL/ HIGH TRIGLY- CERIDES	DIA- BETIC	OVER- WEIGHT	HEALTHY AND I WANT TO STAY THAT WAY	CHECK ALL THAT APPLY TO ME
Eat a wide variety of foods from the DASH Plus Food Lists (*see Food Lists*)	Yes	Yes	Yes	Yes	Yes	Yes	
Avoid refined carbohydrates (foods made with flour, white rice, milled corn) (*see Week 2*)	Yes		Yes	Yes	Yes		
Limit refined carbohydrates (*see Week 2*)		Yes				Yes	
Eat fruits and root vegetables only with other foods, not alone or as snacks (*see Week 3*)			Yes	Yes	Yes		
Avoid partially hydrogenated oils (trans fats) (*see Week 5*)	Yes	Yes	Yes	Yes	Yes	Yes	
Avoid saturated fats (*see Week 5*)	Yes	Yes			Yes		
Limit saturated fats (*see Week 5*)			Yes	Yes		Yes	
Get "good fats" in whole grains, beans and other seeds, seafood (*see Week 5*)	Yes	Yes	Yes	Yes	Yes	Yes	
Eat plenty of leafy greens and other vegetables (*see Week 2*)	Yes	Yes	Yes	Yes	Yes	Yes	

HOW TO USE THIS CHART

YES

Shaded boxes note actions that you should take for various health conditions. To determine which food strategies you need to take, select those conditions that apply to you on the top of the chart and read down the column for specific suggestions.

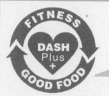

The Healthy Heart Miracle
Personal Roadmap

OTHER STRATEGIES

	NEED TO DO	ALREADY DONE	DOES NOT APPLY TO ME
Stop smoking *(see Week 8)*			
For morbid obesity (over 100 pounds)—Consult with your doctor or healthcare provider *(see Week 8)*			
For chronic inflammation or infection—Consult with your doctor or healthcare provider			
For depression or panic attacks—Consult with your doctor or healthcare provider			
For any other major health issues—Consult with your doctor or healthcare provider			
Recheck abnormal blood tests (check with your doctor for schedule)			
Monitor/log blood pressure daily/weekly/monthly/yearly *(see Week 4)*			
Monitor/log weight loss efforts weekly/monthly/yearly			
Monitor/log weight maintenance monthly/yearly			
Monitor and log muscle gain efforts weekly/monthly/yearly			
Pursue stress-reducing activities			
_____			
_____			
_____			

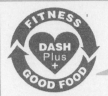

The Healthy Heart Miracle
Personal Roadmap

7

Healthy Heart Strategies for a Loved One

If you are basically healthy but are working to help a loved one (spouse, partner, child, parent, sibling, coworker, friend, etc.), think of yourself as a coach.

Don't try to teach or direct the other person. DO THINGS TOGETHER! What's good for him or her will also be good for you. Concentrate on the Fitness and Food sections in the Personal Roadmap with the other person in mind.

	NEED TO DO	ALREADY DONE	DOES NOT APPLY TO ME
Food Priority Coaching Do you prepare this person's food? ☐ Yes–If yes, go back and use the Personal Roadmap Food Strategies and Specific Food Strategies (see pages 171–172) ☐ No–If no, continue			
If you both live in the same home, but you don't prepare the food: • Volunteer to shop and cook, then start to introduce DASH Plus food and recipes • Find DASH Plus–friendly food sources– Asian markets, restaurants, etc. *(see Week 1)*			
If you don't live together, there may not be much you can do to influence food choices but • Buy "healthy" lunches and snacks to share occasionally • Enlist other friends/coworkers to set good examples • Find carry-out restaurants with good food choices • Set up a "recipe" buddy system where you each try out new DASH Plus recipes, divide in half, and swap recipes			
Fitness Priority Coaching Plan, schedule, carry out all beginner Fitness Program activities together (see beginner's list on page 169). • When you walk, jog, cycle, or work out together, you bring the healthy snacks. • Use the "beginner" or "experienced" Personal Roadmap Worksheets and make notes of ways to make sure each step is followed. • Cater to his/her interests and needs.			

DASH Plus Food Lists

How to Use the Food Lists*

The DASH Plus Food Lists show all the good foods you can choose from—foods that are full of the nutrients you need to keep your heart and body healthy. If you are working to lower your blood pressure or LDL cholesterol, or to control diabetes, choose almost all of your food from these lists. If you are already healthy and want to stay that way, choose about 80 percent of your food from these lists. You can do whatever you like with the other 20 percent.

The symbols next to some of the foods will help you make smart choices to fit your special situation. Here's what they mean:

✳ These are nutrient-rich fruits and root vegetables that contain sugars or starches that cause blood sugar to rise quickly. This is a concern if you are diabetic, have Syndrome X (high triglycerides and low HDL cholesterol), or are trying to lose weight. Eat these fruits and root vegetables only as part of your meal so that the other foods can slow the release of sugars into your bloodstream.

◼ These are nutrient-rich foods that are also concentrated sources of calories. They include seafood, dairy products, nuts, and snack seeds. If you are working to lose weight, lower LDL cholesterol, or control high blood pressure, you need to restrict the portion size of these foods, because they can add a lot of calories without filling you up.

*Note: If your doctor has given you special diet instructions, check with him or her before you incorporate the information in this book into your eating plan. If you have questions about what is appropriate for you, consult your doctor or healthcare provider.

All of the other foods listed have plenty of fiber, so they fill you up; it would be difficult to eat too much of them. Eat as wide a variety of these foods as possible, as often as you like, following the DASH Plus guidelines.

DASH Plus Food Lists

Vegetables (Fresh, Frozen, Canned, or Dried)

Alfalfa sprouts

Artichokes

Arugula

Asparagus

◾ Avocados

Bamboo shoots

Bean sprouts

Beans, green

Beans, lima

Beans, yellow snap

✳ Beets

Broccoli

Brussels sprouts

Cabbage

Cabbage, Chinese

✳ Carrots

Cauliflower

Celery

✳ Celery root

Collard greens

Corn

Cucumbers

Eggplant

Endive

Escarole

Fennel

✳ Jerusalem artichokes

✳ Jicama

✳ = Fruits and Root Vegetables: Eat only with other foods
◾ = Dense Calories/Good Fats: Limit portion sizes

Kohlrabi

Leeks

Lettuce

Mushrooms

Mustard greens

Okra

Onions

* Parsnips

Peas

Peppers

* Potatoes

Pumpkin

Radishes

* Rutabagas

Seaweed, dried

Spinach

Squash

* Sweet potatoes

Swiss chard

Tomatoes

Tomato paste

Tomato sauce

* Turnips

Vegetable-soup mixes

Vegetable soups

Water chestnuts

Watercress

* Yams

* All other root vegetables

All other vegetables

Fruits (Fresh, Frozen, Canned, or Dried)

* Apples

* Apricots

* Asian pears

* Bananas

* Blackberries

* Blueberries

* Carambola (Star Fruit)

* Cherries

* Clementines

◘ Coconut

* Cranberries

* Currants

* Figs

* Grapefruit

* Grapes

* Kiwifruit

Lemons

Limes

* Mangoes

* Melons

* Nectarines

* Oranges

* Peaches

* Pears

* = Fruits and Root Vegetables: Eat only with other foods
◘ = Dense Calories/Good Fats: Limit portion sizes

✳ Pineapple

✳ Plums

✳ Pomegranates

✳ Prunes

✳ Raisins

✳ Raspberries

✳ Rhubarb

✳ Strawberries

✳ Tangerines

✳ Watermelon

✳ All other fruits

Whole Grains

Amaranth

Barley

Buckwheat (Kasha)

Corn, dried

Kashi™ (mixed whole grains)

Millet

Oats

Popcorn (air popped)

Quinoa

Rice, brown

Rye berries

Spelt

Triticale

Wheat berries, all varieties

Wild rice

All other whole grains (seeds)

Breakfast Cereals

All-Bran™

Bran flakes

Cheerios™

Fiber One™

Grape Nuts™

Just Right™

Muesli

Nutri-Grain™

Oat bran

Oatmeal, all styles

Oatmeal Crisp™

Oatmeal Squares™

Puffed wheat

Raisin Bran™

Shredded wheat

Total™

Wheat Chex™

Wheaties™

✳ = Fruits and Root Vegetables: Eat only with other foods
■ = Dense Calories/Good Fats: Limit portion sizes

All other hot whole grain
cereals

All other cold whole grain
or high bran cereals
that meet the criteria on
page 87

Beans, Dried or Canned

Black beans
Black-eyed peas
Broad beans, fava beans
Butter beans
Chickpeas
Chili beans
Garbanzo beans
Great Northern beans
Kidney beans
Lentils
Lima beans
Mung beans

Navy beans
Pink beans
Pinto beans
Red beans
Soybeans
Split peas
White beans
Mixed beans
Bean-soup mixes
Bean-soup cups
All other dried or canned
beans

Nuts and Snack Seeds

◉ Almonds
◉ Brazil nuts
◉ Cashews
   Chestnuts
◉ Coconut
◉ Flaxseeds
◉ Hazelnuts, filberts
◉ Macadamia nuts
◉ Peanuts

◉ Pecans
◉ Pine nuts, piñons, pignoli
◉ Pistachios
◉ Pumpkin seeds
◉ Sunflower seeds
◉ Walnuts
◉ Mixed nuts
◉ All other nuts and snack
seeds

✱ = Fruits and Root Vegetables: Eat only with other foods
◉ = Dense Calories/Good Fats: Limit portion sizes

Soy Products and Other Vegetarian Foods

Soybeans

Soybeans, green (edamame)

◼ Soy nuts, roasted

◼ Texturized Vegetable
    Protein (TVP)

◼ Tofu

◼ Soy milk

◼ Tempeh

◼ Soy burger

◼ Seitan

◼ Vegetable burgers

◼ Almond milk

◼ Rice milk

◼ Other soy meats

◼ Other vegetarian products

Seafood

◼ Bass

◼ Catfish

◼ Clams

◼ Cod

◼ Crab

◼ Flounder

◼ Haddock

◼ Halibut

◼ Herring

◼ Lobster

◼ Mackerel

◼ Mahi mahi

◼ Mussels

◼ Octopus

◼ Oysters

◼ Perch

◼ Pompano

◼ Red snapper

◼ Rockfish

◼ Salmon

◼ Sardines

◼ Scallops

◼ Shrimp

◼ Snapper

◼ Sole

◼ Squid

◼ Surimi

◼ Tilapia

◼ Trout

◼ Tuna

◼ Turbot

◼ All other seafood

✱ = Fruits and Root Vegetables: Eat only with other foods
◼ = Dense Calories/Good Fats: Limit portion sizes

Dairy and Egg Products, Nonfat

- ◼ Milk, nonfat
- ◼ Milk, lactose-free, nonfat
- ◼ Yogurt, nonfat, plain
- ◼ Cottage cheese, nonfat
- ◼ Evaportated milk, nonfat
- ◼ Egg whites
- ◼ Egg substitutes, nonfat
- ◼ Other fat-free dairy products
- ◼ Vegetarian milk substitutes

Fresh Herbs

Basil
Chives
Cilantro, coriander,
   Chinese parsley
Garlic
Gingerroot
Lemongrass
Marjoram

Mint
Oregano
Rosemary
Sage
Tarragon
Thyme
All other fresh herbs

Dried Herbs and Spices

Allspice
Anise
Apple-pie spice mix
Bay leaves
Cajun spice mix
Cayenne pepper
Caraway seeds
Celery seeds
Chili powder

Chinese five-spice powder
Cinnamon
Cloves
Coriander seeds
Cumin seeds
Curry powder
Dill seeds
Fennel seeds
Ginger

✳ = Fruits and Root Vegetables: Eat only with other foods
◼ = Dense Calories/Good Fats: Limit portion sizes

Marjoram

Mustard

Nutmeg

Oregano

Paprika

Pepper, black, crushed red,
red pepper flakes

Poppy seeds

Sage

Sesame seeds

Thyme

Turmeric

All other herb and spices

Seasonings and Condiments

Bean dip

Hoisin sauce

Horseradish

Hot pepper sauce

Ketchup

Liquid smoke

Mustard

Olives

Oyster sauce

Pickles, unsweetened

Salsa

Vanilla extract

Vinegar

Wasabi

Worcestershire sauce

Other seasoning sauces and
condiments

Stock-Up Shopping List

Keep your kitchen stocked with these foods, and you will always be ready to make delicious DASH Plus meals. If you have these items on hand, you will need to shop for fresh produce only once or twice a week.

CANNED BEANS, VEGETABLES, AND FRUITS

- ❑ Black beans
- ❑ Kidney beans
- ❑ Chickpeas
- ❑ Other canned beans of your choice
- ❑ Tomatoes (Italian plum)
- ❑ Tomato sauce
- ❑ Other canned vegetables and fruits of your choice

FROZEN FOODS

- ❑ Corn
- ❑ Peas
- ❑ Green beans
- ❑ Lima beans
- ❑ Pepper-onion mix (chopped green, red, and yellow bell peppers with onions)
- ❑ Veggie burgers and vegetarian meats
- ❑ Other frozen fruits and vegetables of your choice

LONG-KEEPING VEGETABLES AND FRUITS

- ❏ Onions
- ❏ Garlic
- ❏ Carrots
- ❏ Celery
- ❏ Raisins and other dried fruits
- ❏ Other long-keeping fruits and vegetables of your choice

WHOLE GRAINS

- ❏ Barley
- ❏ Wild rice
- ❏ Brown rice
- ❏ Other whole grains of your choice
- ❏ Long-cooking oatmeal, such as Quaker® Old Fashioned Oatmeal
- ❏ Other whole grain breakfast cereals of your choice

CANNED SEAFOOD

- ❏ Tuna
- ❏ Salmon
- ❏ Sardines
- ❏ Other canned seafood of your choice

SPICES, SEASONINGS, AND MISCELLANEOUS ITEMS

- ❏ Bouillon granules or cubes in the flavors of your choice
- ❏ Bottled hot pepper sauce
- ❏ Vinegars: rice, wine, balsamic, etc.
- ❏ Fat-free mayonnaise

❏ Fat-free dressings of your choice
❏ Spices and seasonings of your choice
❏ Nuts and snack seeds of your choice
❏ Shredded or grated cheeses such as Parmesan or Romano

Weekly Menu Plans

The Healthy Heart Miracle
WEEK 1—ASSESSMENT
Menu Plan

FITNESS
DASH
Plus
+
GOOD FOOD

1

For Week 1, Eat and Record Your Typical Diet

	MONDAY	TUESDAY	WEDNESDAY	THURSDAY	FRIDAY	SATURDAY	SUNDAY
B R E A K F A S T							
L U N C H							
D I N N E R							
S N A C K S							

MONDAY	TUESDAY	WEDNESDAY	THURSDAY	FRIDAY	SATURDAY	SUNDAY

**B
R
E
A
K
F
A
S
T**

Oatmeal or other hot whole-grain cereal: Raisins or other dried fruits (optional) • Skim milk, fat-free yogurt, or the milk substitute of your choice on your cereal (optional) • Fresh fruit • Beverage of choice (see below)

**L
U
N
C
H**

Mix and Match Salads: Pick from these choices or others from the recipe on page 200: Salad greens such as romaine lettuce • Your choice of other salad vegetables: tomatoes, avocados, artichoke hearts, red bell peppers • Canned salmon (red sockeye tastes best), canned tuna • Canned beans, canned chickpeas, nuts, peanuts, soy nuts, sunflower seeds, and other seeds • Grated or shredded hard cheese such as Parmesan or Romano • Mild vinegar such as rice wine vinegar and/or low-calorie dressings • Herbs, spices, and spice blends such as Cajun spice blend, salad spice mix, or your personal favorites

**D
I
N
N
E
R**

Mix and Match Salads: Pick from these choices or others from the recipe on page 200: Salad greens such as romaine lettuce • Your choice of other salad vegetables: tomatoes, avocados, artichoke hearts, red bell peppers • Canned salmon (red sockeye taste best), canned tuna • Canned beans, canned chickpeas, nuts, peanuts, soy nuts, sunflower seeds, and other seeds • Grated or shredded hard cheese such as Parmesan or Romano • Mild vinegar such as rice wine vinegar and/or low-calorie dressings • Herbs, spices, and spice blends such as Cajun spice blend, salad spice mix, or your personal favorites

Beverages for all meals and in between: Choose the calorie-free beverage you prefer: water—tap, bottled, sparkling, or flavored • Tea, coffee, calorie-free iced tea, etc.

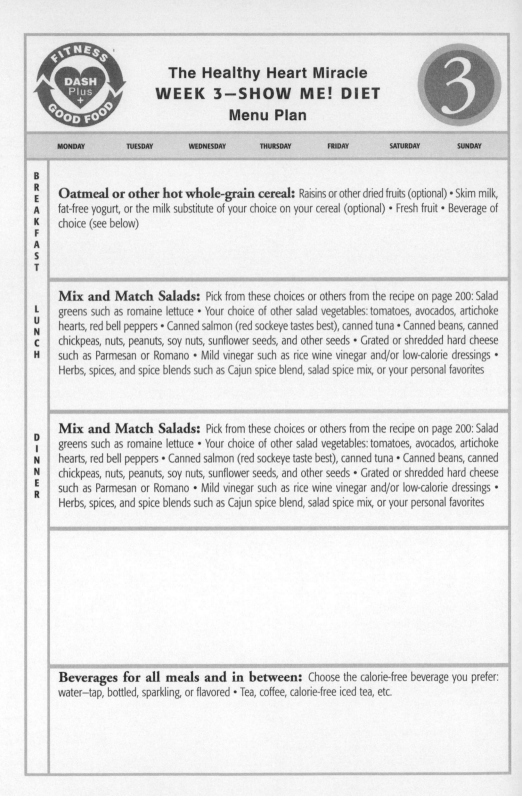

MONDAY	TUESDAY	WEDNESDAY	THURSDAY	FRIDAY	SATURDAY	SUNDAY

BREAKFAST

Oatmeal or other hot whole-grain cereal: Raisins or other dried fruits (optional) • Skim milk, fat-free yogurt, or the milk substitute of your choice on your cereal (optional) • Fresh fruit • Beverage of choice (see below)

LUNCH

Mix and Match Salads: Pick from these choices or others from the recipe on page 200: Salad greens such as romaine lettuce • Your choice of other salad vegetables: tomatoes, avocados, artichoke hearts, red bell peppers • Canned salmon (red sockeye tastes best), canned tuna • Canned beans, canned chickpeas, nuts, peanuts, soy nuts, sunflower seeds, and other seeds • Grated or shredded hard cheese such as Parmesan or Romano • Mild vinegar such as rice wine vinegar and/or low-calorie dressings • Herbs, spices, and spice blends such as Cajun spice blend, salad spice mix, or your personal favorites

DINNER

Mix and Match Salads: Pick from these choices or others from the recipe on page 200: Salad greens such as romaine lettuce • Your choice of other salad vegetables: tomatoes, avocados, artichoke hearts, red bell peppers • Canned salmon (red sockeye taste best), canned tuna • Canned beans, canned chickpeas, nuts, peanuts, soy nuts, sunflower seeds, and other seeds • Grated or shredded hard cheese such as Parmesan or Romano • Mild vinegar such as rice wine vinegar and/or low-calorie dressings • Herbs, spices, and spice blends such as Cajun spice blend, salad spice mix, or your personal favorites

Beverages for all meals and in between: Choose the calorie-free beverage you prefer: water—tap, bottled, sparkling, or flavored • Tea, coffee, calorie-free iced tea, etc.

The Healthy Heart Miracle
WEEK 4*—EASY TO PREPARE
Menu Plan

4

*Recipes in boldface are included in the Recipes section.

	MONDAY	TUESDAY	WEDNESDAY	THURSDAY	FRIDAY	SATURDAY	SUNDAY
BREAKFAST	**Oatmeal or other hot or cold whole-grain cereal:** Raisins or other dried fruits (optional) • Skim milk, fat-free yogurt, or the milk substitute of your choice on your cereal (optional) • Fresh fruit (optional) • Beverage of choice (see below)						
LUNCH	Lentil soup cup Green salad Orange	**Waldorf Salad (L)** Yogurt	**Quick-and-Hearty Chick-pea Soup (L)** Tossed salad Apple	**Extra-Quick Chili (L)** **Banana Rice Pudding**	**Barbecue Beans and Barley (L)** **Quick Coleslaw (L)**	**Hawaiian Smoothie** Bean soup cup	19 Meals Rule-FREE meal. Your choice
DINNER	**Extra-Quick Chili** Brown rice **Waldorf Salad**	**Quick-and-Hearty Chick-pea Soup** Tossed salad Mixed berries	**Mix and Match Salads** **Banana Rice Pudding**	**Barbecue Beans and Barley** **Quick Coleslaw** Watermelon chunks	**Quick Vegetable Curry** Brown rice Strawberries and yogurt	19 Meals Rule-FREE meal. Your choice	**Easy Split-Pea Soup** **Quick Coleslaw (L)**

Snacks: The best DASH Plus snacks are small portions of the good food choices you make for all your meals. If you like munchy-crunchy snacks, try:
- Air-popped popcorn (seasoned with your favorite spice blend, not butter)
- Dry cereal, straight from the box
- Raw vegetables with salsa or bean dip
- Peanut butter on apple slices, celery, or carrots
- Canned sardines, salmon, or tuna with vegetable dippers
Convenient energy sources during prolonged vigorous exercise include trail mixes, dried fruits, or nuts

Beverages for all meals and in between: Choose the calorie-free beverage you prefer: water—tap, bottled, sparkling, or flavored • Tea, coffee, calorie-free iced tea, etc.

Note: (L)=Leftover from previous day
These menus are suggestions to help you plan your meals. Use any of the recipes in this book or your own recipes that contain foods from the Food Lists. More recipes are available at www.healthyheartmiracle.com.

The Healthy Heart Miracle
WEEK 5*—GOOD FATS
Menu Plan

Note: This week's menus are heavy on seafood because I want you to try several new recipes, but feel free to substitute other recipies if you don't want this many seafood dishes.
*Recipes in boldface are included in the Recipes section.

	MONDAY	TUESDAY	WEDNESDAY	THURSDAY	FRIDAY	SATURDAY	SUNDAY
B R E A K F A S T	**Oatmeal or other hot or cold whole-grain cereal:** Raisins or other dried fruits (optional) • Skim milk, fat-free yogurt, or the milk substitute of your choice on your cereal (optional) • Fresh fruit • Beverage of choice (see below).						
L U N C H	Easy Split-Pea Soup (L)	Zesty Crab Salad	Salmon and Corn Bisque (L)	Lentil soup cup	Quick Vegetable Curry (L)	Quick-and-Hearty Chickpea Soup	19 Meals Rule-FREE meal. Your choice
	Tossed salad	Yogurt and bananas	Zesty Crab Salad (L)	Tossed salad	Brown rice (L)	Grapes	
					Tossed Salad		
	Orange			Banana	Peach		
D I N N E R	Shrimp with Wild Rice	Salmon and Corn Bisque	Shrimp with Wild Rice (L)	Quick Vegetable Curry	Baked Fish with Portobello Mushrooms	19 Meals Rule-FREE meal. Your choice	Quick-and-Hearty Chickpea Soup (L)
	Steamed green beans	Steamed baby spinach leaves	Steamed broccoli	Brown rice	Wild rice with dried cherries		Veggie burgers
	Fresh pineapple	Tutti-Frutti Pudding	Bluberries and yogurt	Tutti-Frutti Pudding(L)	Tossed Salad		Sliced tomatoes
					Pineapple Fruit Boats		Blueberries and melon balls

Snacks: The best DASH Plus snacks are small portions of the good food choices you make for all your meals. If you like munchy-crunchy snacks, try:
- Air-popped popcorn (seasoned with your favorite spice blend, not butter)
- Dry cereal, straight from the box
- Raw vegetables with salsa or bean dip
- Peanut butter on apple slices, celery, or carrots
- Canned sardines, salmon, or tuna with vegetable dippers

Convenient energy sources during prolonged vigorous exercise include trail mixes, dried fruits, or nuts.

Beverages for all meals and in between: Choose the calorie-free beverage you prefer: water—tap, bottled, sparkling,or flavored • Tea, coffee, calorie-free iced tea, etc.

Note: (L)=Leftover from previous day
These menus are suggestions to help you plan your meals. Use any of the recipes in this book or your own recipes that contain foods from the Food Lists. More recipes are available at www.healthyheartmiracle.com.

*Recipes in boldface are included in the Recipes section.

	MONDAY	TUESDAY	WEDNESDAY	THURSDAY	FRIDAY	SATURDAY	SUNDAY
B R E A K F A S T	**Oatmeal or other hot or cold whole-grain cereal:** Raisins or other dried fruits (optional) • Skim milk, fat-free yogurt, or the milk substitute of your choice on your cereal (optional) • Fresh fruit • Beverage of choice (see below).						
L U N C H	Bean soup cup	**Dr. Gabe's Famous Eggplant Casserole**	**Chunky Black Bean Soup (L)**	**Catfish Gumbo (L)**	South-western Salad	South-western Salad (L)	19 Meals Rule-FREE meal. Your choice
	Quick Coleslaw	barley (L)	**Almost Instant Spanish Rice(L)**	Tossed salad	Yogurt and blueberries	**Red Pepper Soup (L)**	
		Quick Coleslaw(L)	**Fresh Salsa** Tossed Salad			Banana	
		Apple	Orange				
D I N N E R	**Dr. Gabe's Famous Eggplant Casserole with barley**	**Chunky Black Bean Soup** **Almost Instant Spanish Rice**	**Catfish Gumbo**	**Mix and Match Salads**	**Red Pepper Soup**	19 Meals Rule-FREE meal. Your choice	**Paprika Casserole, barley (L)**
	Strawberries and yogurt	**Fresh Salsa**	Steamed zucchini	**Trail Mix Oatmeal Pudding (L)**	**Paprika Casserole, barley**		Tossed salad
		Easy Banana-Strawberry Sherbet	**Trail Mix Oatmeal Pudding**	Sliced kiwi	Tossed salad Orange wedges		Fresh pineapple with raspberries

Snacks: The best DASH Plus snacks are small portions of the good food choices you make for all your meals. If you like munchy-crunchy snacks, try:
- Air-popped popcorn (seasoned with your favorite spice blend, not butter)
- Dry cereal, straight from the box
- Raw vegetables with salsa or bean dip
- Peanut butter on apple slices, celery, or carrots
- Canned sardines, salmon, or tuna with vegetable dippers

Convenient energy sources during prolonged vigorous exercise include trail mixes, dried fruits, or nuts.

Beverages for all meals and in between: Choose the calorie-free beverage you prefer: water—tap, bottled, sparkling, or flavored • Tea, coffee, calorie-free iced tea, etc.

Note: (L)=Leftover from previous day
These menus are suggestions to help you plan your meals. Use any of the recipes in this book or your own recipes that contain foods from the Food Lists. More recipes are available at www.healthyheartmiracle.com.

*Recipes in boldface are included in the Recipes section.

	MONDAY	TUESDAY	WEDNESDAY	THURSDAY	FRIDAY	SATURDAY	SUNDAY
B R E A K F A S T							

Oatmeal or other hot or cold whole-grain cereal: Raisins or other dried fruits (optional) • Skim milk, fat-free yogurt, or the milk substitute of your choice on your cereal (optional) • Fresh fruit • Beverage of choice (see below).

	MONDAY	TUESDAY	WEDNESDAY	THURSDAY	FRIDAY	SATURDAY	SUNDAY
L U N C H	**Fastest Beans and Rice**	**Hot-and-Sour Mushroom Soup (L)**	**Extra-Quick Chili** with brown rice (L) Tossed salad	**Jamaican Lentil Salad (L)**	**Quick Chickpea Curry (L)**	**Harira (L)**	19 Meals Rule-FREE meal. Your choice
	Fresh Salsa	**Banana Rice Pudding (L)**	Apple	**Almost Instant Spanish Rice**	Brown rice (L)	**Greek Potato Salad (L)**	
	Watermelon			Grapes	Banana	Orange	
D I N N E R	**Hot-and-Sour Mushroom Soup**	**Hummus** with vegetable dippers	**Jamaican Lentil Salad**	**Quick Chickpea Curry** with brown rice	**Harira**	19 Meals Rule-FREE meal. Your choice	**Incredible Creamy Clam Chowder**
	Vietnamese Slaw	**Extra-Quick Chili** with brown rice (L)	Veggie burgers Sliced tomatoes	Mango Chutney, steamed snap peas	**Greek Potato Salad**		**Mix and Match Salads**
	Banana Rice Pudding	Melon balls with mint	Mangos with yogurt	**Indian Rice Pudding**	**Easy Banana-Strawberry Sherbet**		**Fall Fruit Curry**

Snacks: The best DASH Plus snacks are small portions of the good food choices you make for all your meals. If you like munchy-crunchy snacks, try:
- Air-popped popcorn (seasoned with your favorite spice blend, not butter)
- Dry cereal, straight from the box
- Raw vegetables with salsa or bean dip
- Peanut butter on apple slices, celery, or carrots
- Canned sardines, salmon, or tuna with vegetable dippers

Convenient energy sources during prolonged vigorous exercise include trail mixes, dried fruits, or nuts.

Beverages for all meals and in between: Choose the calorie-free beverage you prefer: water—tap, bottled, sparkling, or flavored • Tea, coffee, calorie-free iced tea, etc.

Note: (L)=Leftover from previous day
These menus are suggestions to help you plan your meals. Use any of the recipes in this book or your own recipes that contain foods from the Food Lists. More recipes are available at www.healthyheartmiracle.com.

The Healthy Heart Miracle
WEEK 8*—PARTY BUFFET
Menu Plan

*Recipes in boldface are included in the Recipes section.

Note: This week try all of the featured recipes during the week and select your favorites for a party buffet on Saturday night (or any day of your choice).

	MONDAY	TUESDAY	WEDNESDAY	THURSDAY	FRIDAY	SATURDAY	SUNDAY
BREAKFAST							

BREAKFAST

Oatmeal or other hot or cold whole-grain cereal: Raisins or other dried fruits (optional) • Skim milk, fat-free yogurt, or the milk substitute of your choice on your cereal (optional) • Fresh fruit • Beverage of choice (see below).

	MONDAY	TUESDAY	WEDNESDAY	THURSDAY	FRIDAY	SATURDAY	SUNDAY
LUNCH	Incredible Creamy Clam Chowder (L)	Chafing Dish Chili (L)	Maryland Crab Soup (L)	Smoked Salmon Salad (L)	Penang Shrimp Curry (L)	Mix and Match Salads	19 Meals Rule-FREE meal. Your choice
	Fall Fruit Curry (L)	Fresh Salsa (L)	Fruity Pebbles (L)	Lentil soup cup	Brown rice (L)	Yogurt with raspberries	
					Tossed salad		
		Gingered Fruit Compote (L)		Apple	Banana		

	MONDAY	TUESDAY	WEDNESDAY	THURSDAY	FRIDAY	SATURDAY	SUNDAY
DINNER	Chafing Dish Chili	Maryland Crab Soup	Smoked Salmon Salad	Penang Shrimp Curry with condiments	19 Meals Rule-FREE meal. Your choice	Party buffet: (make any or all) Smoked Salmon Salad, Wild Rice Fruit Salad, Maryland Crab Soup, Sweet Potato Bisque, Chafing Dish Chili, Penang Shrimp Curry, Fruity Pebbles, Gingered Fruit Compote, Fruity Kabobs, Fresh Salsa, Guacamole, Easy Spicy Peanut Dip	Leftovers from party buffet
	Fresh Salsa	Barley	Chafing Dish Chili (L)	Brown rice			
	Guacamole	Tossed salad	Fruity Kabobs	Sliced cucumbers and yogurt			
	Tossed salad						
	Gingered Fruit Compote	Fruity Pebbles		Fresh pineapple			

Snacks: The best DASH Plus snacks are small portions of the good food choices you make for all your meals. If you like munchy-crunchy snacks, try:
- Air-popped popcorn (seasoned with your favorite spice blend, not butter)
- Dry cereal, straight from the box
- Raw vegetables with salsa or bean dip
- Peanut butter on apple slices, celery, or carrots
- Canned sardines, salmon, or tuna with vegetable dippers

Convenient energy sources during prolonged vigorous exercise include trail mixes, dried fruits, or nuts.

Beverages for all meals and in between: Choose the calorie-free beverage you prefer: water—tap, bottled, sparkling, or flavored • Tea, coffee, calorie-free iced tea, etc.

Note: (L)=Leftover from previous day

These menus are suggestions to help you plan your meals. Use any of the recipes in this book or your own recipes that contain foods from the Food Lists. More recipes are available at www.healthyheartmiracle.com.

DASH Plus Recipes

How to Use the DASH Plus Recipes

Following the DASH Plus program may mean changing your cooking style. If cooking your own food is new to you, and some of the recipes in the 8-Week Plan seem daunting, don't get discouraged. Relax! It's hard to go wrong when you cook with fruits, vegetables, whole grains, and beans. You don't need to worry about precise measurements, cooking times, or ingredient preparation. The recipes give you general guidelines, but if you do things a little differently, chances are your dish will still be delicious!

Measurements: Most cooks don't do a lot of measuring. Recipes have to include measurements to give you some idea of what the author has in mind. Measure out a teaspoon of peppercorns and pour it into your hand to see what it looks like; then learn to use your eyes and, of course, your taste buds to measure. I always taste as I go and adjust the seasonings to suit myself. You should do the same.

When a recipe calls for ingredients like an onion, a potato, an orange, or a green pepper, I usually use average-size fruits or vegetables. If you have very small or very large ones on hand, just make a good guess about how much you should use. If you like an ingredient, feel free to add more; if you're not crazy about it, add less, leave it out, or substitute another ingredient (see substitutions).

Chop, Slice, Dice, Mince: Lots of recipes for fruits and vegetables instruct you to cut up the ingredients. How you do that is up to you. If you want to use a food processor or other favorite cutting device, go right ahead. I usually prefer just a knife and chopping board. If the recipe says chop or dice, anything smaller than bite-size is fine. Slice usually means cutting the ingredient crosswise into about ¼-inch pieces. To mince, chop the pieces very small—⅛-inch or so. A garlic press is handy for mincing garlic.

Cooking Times: Cooking times in recipes are approximate; your taste testing is far more important than the clock. Taste a small piece of a carrot or a potato to see if it's tender. Cook the food long enough to blend the flavors but not so long that it turns to mush.

Substitutions: Use the 8-Week Plan recipes as springboards for your own inventions. Be creative! You may want to change a recipe to use up ingredients you have on hand, you may not be able to find an ingredient

Bouillon

Many of the recipes list bouillon in the ingredients. Use your favorite brand of bouillon or experiment with brands until you find some you like. You can use plain water if you wish, but bouillon gives a flavor boost.

Bouillon comes in many forms: cubes, granules, pastes, liquid concentrates that are added to water, and canned bouillons and broths that are ready to use. Follow the package directions to make the amount of bouillon called for in the recipe. Usually you will use one cube or one teaspoon of the product for each cup of water. If a recipe specifies just bouillon granules or bouillon cubes, add them directly to the pot without additional water.

Vegetable- or chicken-flavored bouillons have neutral flavors that go well with any whole grains, beans, or vegetables. Whole grains cooked in vegetable or chicken bouillon can even be used in desserts recipes or as a hot breakfast cereal. Stronger flavored bouillons, such as beef, ham, or fish can be used in hearty recipes such as chilis or soups.

The recipes were tested with bouillon granules that contain salt, and you will find salt in most prepared bouillons. However, low-salt bouillons are available, and if you and your doctor think further salt restriction is advisable, use one of the low-sodium bouillions and adjust the seasonings to your own taste.

in the store, or you may just prefer some other ingredient or seasoning. Make a note of the substitutions you've used when you like the results.

Try New Foods: Be brave about trying foods you've never liked before. New combinations and seasonings can change your mind. If I've tried an ingredient three different ways and still don't like it, I cross it off my list.

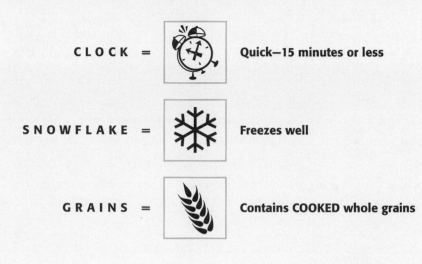

CLOCK =   Quick—15 minutes or less

SNOWFLAKE =   Freezes well

GRAINS =   Contains COOKED whole grains

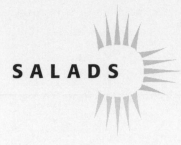

SALADS

Mix and Match Salads · · · · · · · · · · · · · · · · · · ·

3 SERVINGS

Mix and Match Salads are whole meals in a bowl. Start with any lettuce or salad greens you like, and add ANY other ingredients from the Food Lists on pages 177–183. Try to get several different bright colors in the bowl, including something red, orange, or yellow. Here's one of my favorite combinations.

*2 Romaine lettuce hearts, sliced crosswise into ½-inch strips,
   or torn into bite-size pieces*
1 (10-ounce) box grape or cherry tomatoes
1 (6-ounce) jar marinated artichoke hearts, drained
1 ripe avocado, cut in ½-inch chunks
1 red bell pepper, cut in ¼-inch strips
1 (3-ounce) can red sockeye salmon
¼ cup shredded Romano cheese
1 teaspoon Cajun spice blend, or to taste
2 tablespoons rice vinegar or light wine vinegar

Toss all the ingredients together in a salad bowl and serve.

Nutritional Analysis

CALORIES: 277, CARBOHYDRATES: 16G, FIBER: 7G, TOTAL FAT: 19G,
SATURATED FAT: 5G, PROTEIN: 14G

Note: This is just one of the endless combinations. Start with 3 to 4 cups of salad greens per person. Then add whatever amount you like of the foods from the Vegetables, Fruits, Whole Grains, Beans, Vegetarian Products, and Spices and Seasonings Food Lists (pages 177–183).

The DASH Plus guidelines explain the few ingredients that need to have limited portion sizes:

Seafood—maximum of 6 ounces (two 3-ounce servings) per day
Cheese—maximum of 3 servings per day; 1 ounce of dry (low-fat)
    cheese counts as 1 dairy serving
Nuts and Seeds—maximum of ¼ cup (two 2-tablesoon servings)
    per day
Up to 1 tablespoon of olive oil per day in your dressing if you like;
    otherwise, use plain vinegar or a low-calorie bottled dressing

To make Mix and Match Salad preparation even easier, prepare a batch of Salad-Starter Vegetables from the recipe below.

Salad-Starter Vegetables

NUMBER OF SERVINGS DEPENDS ON QUANTITY OF
VEGETABLES USED

Some salad vegetables can be cut up in advance because they will keep well for several days, others wilt quickly and should be cut up just before you use them. You can prepare a large quantity of salad-starter vegetables and refrigerate them for a whole week's worth of Mix and Match Salads. They're also good for munching as a quick snack.

Prepare any or all of the following:

raw cauliflower, broken in florets
raw broccoli, broken in florets
sliced carrots
sliced or chopped celery
sliced radishes
sliced green onions
canned chickpeas, drained
red or green cabbage, thinly sliced
1 to 2 tablespoons rice vinegar (optional)

Combine the vegetables in a large container with a tight-fitting lid. Toss them with a tablespoon or two of rice vinegar, or other light vinegar if you wish. Use some for today's salad and store the rest to use over the next several days.

Nutritional Analysis

ALL SALAD-STARTER VEGETABLES ARE VERY LOW IN CALORIES AND FAT. THEY ARE ALSO HIGH IN FIBER.

Banana-Shrimp Salad . . . .
4 SERVINGS

1 pound small shrimp, steamed and peeled
1 cup chopped celery
1 red bell pepper, chopped
1 cup baby carrots, sliced crosswise
1 (10-ounce) bag baby spinach leaves
½ cup chopped cilantro or Italian parsley leaves

1 tablespoon lime juice
1 teaspoon grated lime rind
¼ cup rice vinegar
1 teaspoon ground cumin
Pinch of cayenne pepper, or to taste
4 ripe bananas, sliced
½ cup chopped nuts (your choice: macadamias, cashews,
  pecans, peanuts, or whatever else you like)

Combine all the ingredients except the bananas and nuts, mix well, and chill. When ready to serve, gently stir in the bananas and sprinkle the nuts on top.

Nutritional Analysis

CALORIES: 378, CARBOHYDRATES: 43G, FIBER: 10G, TOTAL FAT: 11G, SATURATED FAT: 2G, PROTEIN: 33G

Note: You can buy shrimp already steamed and peeled, but they're very easy to make yourself. One of the best ways to cook the shrimp is in the countertop steamer I recommend for cooking whole grains. Check your instruction manual for directions.

Greek Potato Salad

6 SERVINGS

2 pounds (about 6) medium red potatoes or baby potatoes,
  unpeeled
2 (6-ounce) jars marinated artichoke hearts, drained
½ cup chopped celery
¼ cup chopped onion

½ cup plain nonfat yogurt
¼ cup Dijon mustard
Juice of 1 lemon
1 teaspoon dried oregano
Pinch of cayenne pepper, or more to taste
Freshly ground black pepper, to taste

Boil the potatoes until just tender, about 20 minutes for medium potatoes, 10 to 15 minutes for baby potatoes. Drain the water, then cut into bite-size pieces. Combine the potatoes with the remaining ingredients and chill at least 30 minutes.

Nutritional Analysis

CALORIES: 300, CARBOHYDRATES: 59G, FIBER: 7G, TOTAL FAT: 6G, SATURATED FAT: 1G, PROTEIN: 8G

Jamaican Lentil Salad

4 SERVINGS

1 cup tiny green lentils (French style or le Puy)
2 garlic cloves, minced
6 cups bouillon (see page 198)
1 small sweet onion, chopped
1 celery stalk, chopped
1 (10-ounce) box grape or cherry tomatoes, halved or
  quartered if large
1 bunch radishes, sliced
1 cup baby carrots, sliced crosswise
¼ cup chopped Italian parsley leaves
Juice of 1 lime

¼ cup rice vinegar, or to taste
Bottled hot pepper sauce, to taste

Bring the lentils, garlic, and bouillon to a boil and simmer until the lentils are tender but not mushy, about 20 minutes. Place the lentils in a colander, rinse with cold water, and let them drain. Combine the lentils with the remaining ingredients and chill until ready to serve.

Nutritional Analysis

CALORIES: 231, CARBOHYDRATES: 40G, FIBER: 14G, TOTAL FAT: 2G, SATURATED FAT: 1G, PROTEIN: 17G

Note: This salad is supposed to be quite spicy. Whenever you're not sure about your guests' tastes, make the dish tame and place the bottle of hot sauce on the side so your guests can customize their food to suit their tastes.

Quick Coleslaw . . . .

4 SERVINGS

1 small head cabbage, thinly sliced
1 red or green bell pepper, finely chopped
2 teaspoons caraway seeds
¼ cup rice vinegar
¼ cup nonfat mayonnaise

Combine all the ingredients. Serve the slaw immediately or refrigerate for later.

Nutritional Analysis

CALORIES: 77, CARBOHYDRATES: 16G, FIBER: 6G, TOTAL FAT: 1G, SATURATED FAT: 0G, PROTEIN: 4G

Note: Rice vinegar is a mild vinegar that you can use straight from the bottle for cooking or to dress salads. It's often found in the Asian section of supermarkets, or it may be stocked with the other vinegars. If you can't find it, substitute any mild vinegar.

Smoked Salmon Salad

4 SERVINGS

½ pound smoked salmon, cut in bite-size pieces
1 (16-ounce) can small white beans, drained and rinsed
1 small sweet onion, chopped
2 celery stalks, chopped
1 cup frozen green peas, defrosted
½ cup chopped Italian parsley leaves
1 teaspoon dried oregano
Juice of 1 lemon
¼ cup rice vinegar, or to taste
Pinch of cayenne pepper, or dash of bottled hot pepper sauce,
  or to taste
Romaine lettuce (optional)

Combine all the ingredients and chill. When ready to serve, arrange the salad on a bed of lettuce leaves, if desired.

Nutritional Analysis
CALORIES: 165, CARBOHYDRATES: 28G, FIBER: 8G, TOTAL FAT: 1G,
SATURATED FAT: 0G, PROTEIN: 10G

Southwestern Salad for Don Imus

6 SERVINGS

2 cups cooked brown rice or barley
1 (16-ounce) can black beans or kidney beans, drained and
* rinsed*
2 cups cooked corn kernels (fresh or frozen)
1 red bell pepper, chopped
1 small onion, chopped
¼ cup rice vinegar, or more to taste
¼ cup chopped cilantro leaves
1 minced jalapeño chile, or cayenne pepper to taste
1 tablespoon chili powder

Combine all the ingredients. This dish tastes even better if you let it stand, refrigerated or at room temperature, for one hour before serving.

Nutritional Analysis
CALORIES: 195, CARBOHYDRATES: 40G, FIBER: 7G, TOTAL FAT: 2G,
SATURATED FAT: 0G, PROTEIN: 8G

Note: Salads don't freeze well because the crispy vegetables will turn mushy. Most will keep for several days in the refrigerator. This salad and many of the other whole-grain salads taste even better the second day when the flavors have blended. They're great for packing in lunches.

Vietnamese Slaw

4 SERVINGS

> 4 cups shredded Napa or Chinese cabbage
> 1 cup shredded carrots
> ½ cup thinly sliced sweet onion
> 2 cups canned pineapple chunks, drained
> ¼ cup rice vinegar
> ¼ cup chopped cilantro leaves
> ½ cup chopped peanuts

Combine all the ingredients except the peanuts. Chill if preparing ahead. Sprinkle with the chopped peanuts before serving.

Nutritional Analysis

CALORIES: 180, CARBOHYDRATES: 21G, FIBER: 6G, TOTAL FAT: 10G, SATURATED FAT: 1G, PROTEIN: 7G

Note: Pre-cut or baby vegetables, such as shredded or baby carrots, are more expensive than bulk ones, but the convenience is worth the cost to many busy people.

Waldorf Salad

6 SERVINGS

> 4 crisp apples, cored and diced
> 2 tablespoons lemon juice
> 1 cup chopped celery
> 1 cup raisins
> ½ cup chopped pecans or walnuts

1 teaspoon curry powder (optional)
2 tablespoons rice vinegar
½ cup nonfat mayonnaise

Toss the apples in the lemon juice, then mix with the remaining ingredients. To prepare the salad ahead of time, combine everything except the mayonnaise, cover, and chill. Stir in the mayonnaise just before serving.

Nutritional Analysis

CALORIES: 218, CARBOHYDRATES: 42G, FIBER: 5G, TOTAL FAT: 6G, SATURATED FAT: IG, PROTEIN: 4G

Note: I never peel fruits or vegetables unless the skins are too tough, thick, or bitter to eat. Vitamins, minerals, phytochemicals, and fiber are often concentrated in or near the skin. So don't throw them away if they're edible! The "wax" used to coat some fruits and vegetables is harmless. Just rinse or scrub and enjoy.

Wild Rice Fruit Salad

8 SERVINGS

4 cups cooked wild rice
1 cup golden raisins
1 green bell pepper, chopped
2 cups seedless grapes
1 bunch green onions, sliced (white part only)
½ cup chopped Italian parsley leaves
¼ cup lemon juice
2 teaspoons mild curry powder
½ cup nonfat mayonnaise, or enough to moisten the grains

Combine all the ingredients. If you make this ahead of time, stir in the mayonnaise just before serving.

Nutritional Analysis

CALORIES: 170, CARBOHYDRATES: 40G, FIBER: 3G, TOTAL FAT: 1G, SATURATED FAT: 0G, PROTEIN: 4G

Note: Bottled lemon juice is available in supermarkets and is a great convenience. It tastes like fresh juice when you use it in recipes.

Zesty Crab Salad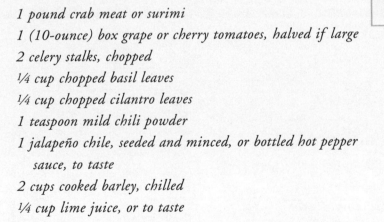

6 SERVINGS

1 pound crab meat or surimi
1 (10-ounce) box grape or cherry tomatoes, halved if large
2 celery stalks, chopped
¼ cup chopped basil leaves
¼ cup chopped cilantro leaves
1 teaspoon mild chili powder
1 jalapeño chile, seeded and minced, or bottled hot pepper
*   sauce, to taste*
2 cups cooked barley, chilled
¼ cup lime juice, or to taste

Combine all the ingredients and serve, or chill for later.

Nutritional Analysis

CALORIES: 199, CARBOHYDRATES: 24G, FIBER: 6G, TOTAL FAT: 2G, SATURATED FAT: 0G, PROTEIN: 21G

Note: Many of these recipes assume you have cooked whole grains on hand in your freezer or refrigerator. To start building up your stock, see page 82.

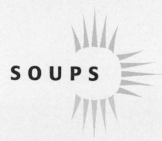

SOUPS

Chunky Black Bean Soup

6 SERVINGS

> 2 onions, chopped
> 4 garlic cloves, minced
> 4 carrots, chopped
> 2 celery stalks, chopped
> 1 green bell pepper, chopped
> 1 jalapeño chile, seeded and minced, or pinch of cayenne
>   pepper, or to taste
> 2 teaspoons ground cumin
> 2 cups bouillon (see page 198)
> 2 (16-ounce) cans black beans, undrained
> 1 (16-ounce) can tomatoes, undrained and chopped
> Chopped cilantro leaves for garnish (optional)

Combine the onions, garlic, carrots, celery, bell pepper, jalapeño, cumin, and bouillon in a large pot. Bring to a boil, reduce the heat and simmer uncovered 15 to 20 minutes, or until the vegetables are soft. Add the beans and tomatoes and simmer 15 to 20 minutes more. Serve sprinkled with chopped cilantro, if desired.

Nutritional Analysis

CALORIES: 237, CARBOHYDRATES: 42G, FIBER: 13G, TOTAL FAT: 4G,
SATURATED FAT: IG, PROTEIN: 12G

Note: Any black bean soup can be dressed up with a dollop of yogurt,
salsa (page 245), or guacamole (page 246).

Easy Split-Pea Soup

6 SERVINGS

> *8 cups bouillon (see page 198)*
> *1 onion, chopped*
> *2 garlic cloves, minced*
> *2 teaspoons curry powder*
> *2 teaspoons ground cumin*
> *1 teaspoon ground cinnamon*
> *Pinch of cayenne pepper, or to taste*
> *1 pound yellow split peas*

Bring ½ cup of the bouillon to a boil in a large pot, stir in the onion, garlic, curry, cumin, cinnamon, and cayenne and cook for 5 minutes. Add
the peas, bring to a boil, and cook for about 1 hour, or until the split peas
are soft. Puree with a hand blender, if you wish, to make it very smooth.

Nutritional Analysis

CALORIES: 257, CARBOHYDRATES: 42G, FIBER: 16G, TOTAL FAT: 2G,
SATURATED FAT: OG, PROTEIN: 42G

Note: This recipe, and many others in the soup section, takes more than
15 minutes to make, so they don't qualify as "Quick." But you just dump

everything into a pot and let it cook by itself, which certainly makes it "Easy."

Harira ·

6 SERVINGS

1 large onion, chopped
1 red bell pepper, chopped
2 celery stalks, chopped
2 garlic cloves, chopped
8 cups bouillon (see page 198)
1 cup lentils
1 (28-ounce) can Italian plum tomatoes, undrained and
*   chopped*
½ teaspoon Harissa Sauce (page 247) or hot pepper sauce, to
*   taste*
1 can chickpeas, undrained
½ cup chopped Italian parsley leaves
¼ cup lemon juice, or more to taste
Lemon wedges for garnish
Freshly ground black pepper, to taste

Combine the onion, bell pepper, celery, and garlic in ½ cup of bouillon in a large pot and cook until softened, 5 to 10 minutes. Stir in the lentils and the remaining bouillon and bring to a boil. Reduce the heat to a simmer, add the tomatoes and harissa, and cook until the lentils are tender, 25 to 30 minutes. Add the chickpeas, parsley, and lemon juice. If you wish, stir in a cup or two of cooked whole grains or place ½ cup of grains in the bottom of each serving bowl. Serve with lemon wedges and season with black pepper.

Nutritional Analysis

CALORIES: 235, CARBOHYDRATES: 39G, FIBER: 13G, TOTAL FAT: 3G,
SATURATED FAT: 0G, PROTEIN: 16G

Hot-and-Sour Mushroom Soup. . . . .

4 SERVINGS

6 cups bouillon (see page 198)
One 6-inch piece lemongrass, split lengthwise and crushed
  (optional)
Zest of 1 lemon, grated
2 garlic cloves, minced
1 (6-ounce) can bamboo shoots, cut into matchsticks
5 green onions, sliced thin (white part only)
1 pound mushrooms, cleaned and sliced
2 tablespoons oyster sauce (optional; see Note)
2 tablespoons cornstarch
2 tablespoons water
Juice of 1 lemon
Pinch of cayenne pepper, or to taste
¼ cup chopped cilantro or Italian parsley leaves

In a large pot, bring the bouillon, lemongrass, lemon zest, and garlic to a
boil. Reduce the heat and simmer, covered, 15 to 20 minutes. Add the
bamboo shoots, green onions, mushrooms, and oyster sauce, if desired,
and cook 5 minutes. Mix the cornstarch and water into a smooth paste,
stir it into the soup, and return the soup to a boil. Remove the lemongrass
and stir in the lemon juice and cayenne pepper. Ladle into soup bowls and
garnish with the cilantro.

Nutritional Analysis

CALORIES: 112, CARBOHYDRATES: 18G, FIBER: 3G, TOTAL FAT: 2G,
SATURATED FAT: 1G, PROTEIN: 9G

Note: Lemongrass is available in many Asian markets and in some specialty stores. It's tough, so don't eat it. Use it to give a special lemony flavor to soup or tea. If you can't find it, the recipe is still delicious without it.

Oyster sauce, hoisin sauce, and many other interesting seasonings can be found in the Asian food section of large supermarkets. If you live in an area that has Asian markets, you'll find a much wider variety there. Don't be afraid to experiment!

Incredible Creamy Clam Chowder

4 SERVINGS

1 large onion, chopped
6 cups bouillon (see page 198)
1 medium cauliflower, cut into chunks
1 cup quick-cooking or rolled oats
1 teaspoon dried oregano
Pinch of cayenne pepper, or to taste
1 (6.5-ounce) can chopped clams, undrained
Freshly ground black pepper, to taste
Chopped chives or parsley for garnish (optional)

Combine the onion, bouillon, cauliflower, oats, oregano, and cayenne pepper in a large pot and bring to a boil. Reduce the heat and simmer gently for 60 minutes, uncovered, stirring occasionally. Using a hand blender, puree until smooth. Stir in the clams and their juice, and adjust the seasonings. Season with black pepper and garnish with chives or parsley, if desired.

Nutritional Analysis

CALORIES: 214, CARBOHYDRATES: 26G, FIBER: 5G, TOTAL FAT: 3G,
SATURATED FAT: 1G, PROTEIN: 22G

Note: You can blend any soup in a regular blender, but it's a nuisance. Make a small investment in a hand blender if you don't have one. You won't believe how many delicious, creamy soups you can make using a hand blender, all without adding any cream or butter.

Maryland Crab Soup . . . .

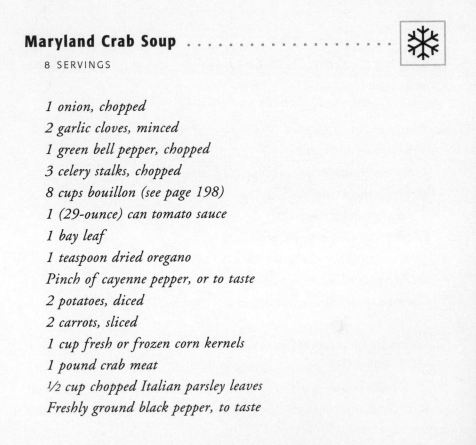

8 SERVINGS

1 onion, chopped
2 garlic cloves, minced
1 green bell pepper, chopped
3 celery stalks, chopped
8 cups bouillon (see page 198)
1 (29-ounce) can tomato sauce
1 bay leaf
1 teaspoon dried oregano
Pinch of cayenne pepper, or to taste
2 potatoes, diced
2 carrots, sliced
1 cup fresh or frozen corn kernels
1 pound crab meat
½ cup chopped Italian parsley leaves
Freshly ground black pepper, to taste

Combine the onions, garlic, bell pepper, celery, and ½ cup of the bouillon in a large pot and cook until softened, 5 to 10 minutes. Add the remaining bouillon, tomato sauce, bay leaf, oregano, cayenne pepper, potatoes, and carrots, and cook until the potatoes are tender, about 20 minutes. Stir in the corn, crabmeat, and parsley, and simmer 5 minutes. Season with black pepper.

Nutritional Analysis

CALORIES: 178, CARBOHYDRATES: 25G, FIBER: 4G, TOTAL FAT: 2G, SATURATED FAT: 0G, PROTEIN: 18G

Note: This is my favorite soup. You can make it with any seafood. If you're a vegetarian, omit the crab, and you'll have a great vegetable soup.

Quick-and-Hearty Chickpea Soup . . . .

6 SERVINGS

½ cup bulgur
6 cups bouillon (see page 198)
2 (16-ounce) cans chickpeas, undrained
2 teaspoons dried oregano
¼ teaspoon Harissa Sauce (see page 247), or hot pepper sauce, to taste
1 (10-ounce) bag baby spinach leaves
Lemon slices or wedges for garnish

Bring the bulgur and bouillon to a boil in a large pot. Add the chickpeas, oregano, and Harissa Sauce or hot pepper sauce. Return to a boil, reduce the heat, and simmer until the bulgur is soft, 5 to 10 minutes. Puree with a hand blender to make a chunky soup. Stir in the spinach leaves and serve with lemon wedges.

Nutritional Analysis

CALORIES: 220, CARBOHYDRATES: 35G, FIBER: 12G, TOTAL FAT: 4G,
SATURATED FAT: 0G, PROTEIN: 11G

Red Pepper Soup

6 SERVINGS

6 cups bouillon (see page 198)
1 onion, chopped
4 garlic cloves, minced
2 celery stalks, chopped
4 red bell peppers, cut in chunks
1 pound red potatoes, cut in chunks
1 tablespoon chili powder
Pinch of cayenne pepper or a few drops of bottled hot pepper
  sauce, to taste

Combine all the ingredients in a large pot. Bring to a boil, reduce the heat, and simmer until the vegetables are very soft, 30 to 40 minutes. Blend with a hand blender until smooth. Adjust the seasonings and serve.

Nutritional Analysis

CALORIES: 117, CARBOHYDRATES: 23G, FIBER: 4G, TOTAL FAT: 1G,
SATURATED FAT: 0G, PROTEIN: 6G

Note: Why would you want to make such a big pot of soup if you have only one or two people to cook for? Because it's just as much work to make one serving as it is to make 10, so you might as well stock up! Cook the whole batch and freeze the leftovers. Soon you'll have a whole supply of your own fast foods. Double your favorite recipes to save even more time.

Salmon and Corn Bisque

6 SERVINGS

1 onion, chopped

4 cups bouillon (see page 198)

2 medium red potatoes, cut into ½-inch chunks

1 teaspoon dried oregano

¼ teaspoon dried thyme

Pinch of cayenne pepper, or to taste

½ cup dry rolled or quick-cooking oats

½ cup chopped red bell pepper

1 pound salmon steak or fillet, skinned and cut into 1- to
*   2-inch chunks*

2 cups frozen or fresh corn

Freshly ground black pepper, to taste

Paprika for garnish (optional)

Combine the onion, bouillon, potatoes, oregano, thyme, cayenne pepper, and oatmeal in a large pot. Bring to a boil, reduce the heat, and simmer, uncovered, until the potatoes are just tender, 15 to 20 minutes. Puree briefly with a hand blender until chunky. Add the red bell pepper and raise the heat just enough to return the soup to a boil. Stir in the salmon and corn, reduce the heat, and simmer until the largest salmon chunks are opaque in the center, about 5 minutes. Ladle into bowls and season with black pepper and a pinch of paprika, if desired.

Nutritional Analysis

CALORIES: 300, CARBOHYDRATES: 44G, FIBER: 7G, TOTAL FAT: 5G, SATURATED FAT: 1G, PROTEIN: 24G

Sweet Potato Bisque ·

6 SERVINGS

1 onion, chopped

2 celery stalks, chopped

3 pounds sweet potatoes, peeled and diced

8 cups bouillon (see page 198)

1 tablespoon mild curry powder

2 teaspoons dried thyme

1 teaspoon freshly ground black or white pepper

Pinch of cayenne pepper, or to taste

¼ cup brandy (optional)

2 cups light coconut milk or soy milk

Combine the onion, celery, sweet potatoes, bouillon, curry powder, thyme, and ground peppers in a large pot. Bring to a boil, reduce the heat, and simmer until the potatoes are soft, 30 to 40 minutes. With a slotted spoon, remove about 2 cups of the vegetables and set aside. Puree the remaining soup with a hand blender until fairly smooth. Return the vegetables to the pot, stir in the brandy, if desired, and coconut or soy milk, and heat through.

Nutritional Analysis

CALORIES: 328, CARBOHYDRATES: 61G, FIBER: 6G, TOTAL FAT: 3G, SATURATED FAT: 1G, PROTEIN: 10G

Three Sisters Soup . . . .

10 SERVINGS

3 pounds winter squash, such as acorn or Hubbard

3 cups bouillon (see page 198)

3 onions, chopped

3 teaspoons mild chili powder

Pinch of cayenne, or to taste

3 (16-ounce) cans white beans, undrained

3 cups fresh or frozen lima beans

3 cups frozen corn kernels

3 tablespoons chopped chives or green onions (optional)

Pierce the squash with a knife several times. Set in a microwave-safe dish and microwave on high for 3 minutes. When cool enough to handle, cut the squash in half and scoop out the seeds. Return the squash to the microwave and cook until tender, about 5 minutes more. Remove the skin and cut the squash into bite-size chunks.

Meanwhile, bring ½ cup of the bouillon to a boil in a large pot, add the onions, and cook 5 to 10 minutes. Stir in the rest of the bouillon, the chili powder, cayenne, and white beans. Simmer gently until the squash is ready. Stir the squash into the soup. Lightly mash the beans and squash to thicken the soup, or use a hand blender. Add the lima beans and simmer 10 minutes. Stir in the corn, then ladle the soup into bowls, and garnish with chopped chives or green onions, if desired.

Nutritional Analysis

CALORIES: 320, CARBOHYDRATES: 62G, FIBER: 15G, TOTAL FAT: 1G, SATURATED FAT: 0G, PROTEIN: 18G

Note: The "Three Sisters" are corn, beans, and squash, which were grown together by Native Americans. The beans climbed on the corn stalks and returned nitrogen to the soil, and the low-growing squash vines shaded all the roots and kept weeds from sprouting. They can all be combined in one pot of delicious soup—using a recipe that calls for three of everything!

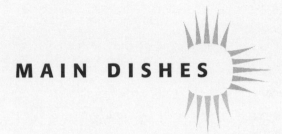

MAIN DISHES

Baked Fish with Portobello Mushrooms

4 SERVINGS

2 Vidalia or other sweet onions, sliced
4 to 6 salmon steaks, or any fish of your choice
1 pound portobello mushrooms, sliced
Juice of 1 lemon
Fresh herbs of your choice (optional)
Freshly ground black pepper, to taste
Lemon wedges for garnish

Preheat the oven to 350 degrees. Place a layer of onion slices on the bottom of a casserole dish large enough to hold the fish steaks in one or two layers. Place the fish steaks on the onions, then arrange the mushrooms and remaining onion slices on top. (If you are using two layers of fish, place some of the mushrooms and onions between the layers and the remaining ones on top.) Lay the fresh herbs on top, if you are using them, and squeeze the lemon juice over all. Cover tightly and bake until the fish is opaque in the middle (test with a knife or fork), about 30 minutes. Season with pepper and serve with lemon wedges.

Nutritional Analysis

CALORIES: 298, CARBOHYDRATES: 21G, FIBER: 7G, TOTAL FAT: 2G, SATURATED FAT: 0G, PROTEIN: 51G

Note: Portobello mushrooms are large, meaty, and delicious. If you can't find them, substitute regular button mushrooms.

Barbecue Beans and Barley

8 SERVINGS

1 onion, chopped
2 garlic cloves, minced
1 (12-ounce) can beer or 1½ cups water
½ cup ketchup
*½ cup brown sugar (diabetics can use an artificial sweetener
    to taste)*
2 tablespoons Worcestershire sauce
½ teaspoon liquid smoke, or to taste
½ teaspoon ground cinnamon
2 (16-ounce) cans pink beans, drained
2 cups cooked barley

Combine the onion, garlic, beer, ketchup, brown sugar, Worcestershire sauce, liquid smoke, and cinnamon in a large pot. Bring to a boil and cook gently until thickened, about 10 minutes. Stir in the beans and barley, return to a boil, then reduce the heat and simmer for 10 minutes.

Nutritional Analysis

CALORIES: 330, CARBOHYDRATES: 68G, FIBER: 10G, TOTAL FAT: 1G,
SATURATED FAT: 0G, PROTEIN: 13G

Note: You'll find bottles of liquid smoke in the spice section of your
supermarket.

Catfish Gumbo . . . .

6 SERVINGS

6 cups bouillon (see page 198)
1 large onion, chopped
4 garlic cloves, minced
1 green bell pepper, chopped
2 celery stalks, sliced
1 (28-ounce) can Italian plum tomatoes, undrained and
* chopped*
2 teaspoons dried oregano
Pinch of cayenne, or to taste
3 cups fresh or frozen okra or green beans, cut into bite-size
* pieces*
1 pound catfish fillets, cut into 1-inch pieces
1 cup frozen corn
¼ cup chopped Italian parsley leaves for garnish
Cooked whole grains of your choice
Bottled hot pepper sauce (optional)

Bring ½ cup of the bouillon to a boil in a large pot. Add the onion, garlic,
bell pepper, and celery and cook until softened, about 5 minutes. Add the
remaining bouillon, the tomatoes, oregano, and cayenne, bring to a boil,
and cook 5 to 10 minutes. Stir in the okra or green beans and simmer 5

minutes. Return the soup to a boil and stir in the catfish. Reduce the heat and simmer until the fish is opaque and the vegetables are tender, about 5 minutes. Stir in the corn. Serve the gumbo over a mound of whole grains and garnish with the parsley. Pass the hot pepper sauce, if desired.

Nutritional Analysis

CALORIES: 220, CARBOHYDRATES: 33G, FIBER: 7G, TOTAL FAT: 3G, SATURATED FAT: 1G, PROTEIN: 18G

Note: Different types of fish are interchangeable in most of my recipes, so use whatever is on sale or looks good at the seafood counter.

Chafing Dish Chili . . . .

8 SERVINGS

2 large onions, chopped
2 green bell peppers, chopped
4 garlic cloves, chopped
3 tablespoons mild chili powder
1 tablespoon ground cumin
1/2 teaspoon ground cinnamon
1/4 teaspoon cayenne pepper, or to taste
5 cups bouillon (see page 198)
1 pound green lentils
1 cup uncooked bulgur
1 (28-ounce) cans Italian plum tomatoes, undrained, and
   chopped

Optional garnishes
Fat-free sour cream
Fresh Salsa (page 245, or in a jar)

Chopped cilantro
Slivers of red, green, and yellow bell pepper
Guacamole (page 246)
Cooked whole grains
Bottled hot pepper sauce

Combine all the ingredients in a large pot, bring to a boil, and simmer, stirring occasionally, until the lentils are tender, 30 to 40 minutes. Turn off the heat and let the chili sit until ready to serve. (You can also make this dish ahead and refrigerate it.)

Just before serving, reheat and transfer to a chafing dish or other buffet serving dish. Surround with mugs or small bowls with handles. Top the chili with your choice of garnishes, if desired.

Nutritional Analysis
CALORIES: 330, CARBOHYDRATES: 64G, FIBER: 16G, TOTAL FAT: 1G, SATURATED FAT: 0G, PROTEIN: 21G

Crab Delight . . . .
4 SERVINGS

Juice of 1 lemon
1 red bell pepper, chopped
4 green onions, minced
2 tablespoons grated fresh gingerroot
2 tomatoes, chopped
¼ pound mushrooms, chopped
1 (8-ounce) can water chestnuts, diced
1 cup broccoli florets
¼ pound snow peas

1 pound crabmeat or surimi
Freshly ground black pepper, to taste
Cooked brown rice (optional)

In a medium saucepan, cook the bell pepper, onions, and gingerroot in the lemon juice until softened, about 5 minutes. Add the tomatoes, mushrooms, water chestnuts, and broccoli; cover and steam until the broccoli is crisp-tender, about 10 minutes. Add the snow peas and crabmeat and cook 2 to 3 minutes. Season with black pepper and serve over brown rice, if desired. This dish is good chilled for lunch the next day, too.

Nutritional Analysis

CALORIES: 296, CARBOHYDRATES: 42G, FIBER: 8G, TOTAL FAT: 3G, SATURATED FAT: 1G, PROTEIN: 27G

Note: This and many other recipes are very quick if you have cooked whole grains on hand. That's why I always recommend cooking a pound at a time and freezing the leftovers. Packaged instant brown rice is another solution, but I find the texture too mushy. Instant barley is better and takes only 10 minutes to prepare, so it's a good solution. Instant barley is often placed in the cereal section of supermarkets because it's from Quaker Oats. Look for a yellow box. (Their regular barley box is white.)

Extra-Quick Chili

6 SERVINGS

1 (16-ounce) bag frozen onion-pepper mix
2 garlic cloves, minced
1 (28-ounce) can Italian plum tomatoes, cut in pieces
1 bouillon cube
1 tablespoon mild chili powder

Pinch of cayenne pepper, or to taste
2 (16-ounce) cans kidney beans or black beans, undrained
Cooked whole grains of your choice (optional)

Combine all the ingredients except the grains in a large pot, bring to a boil, and simmer 5 to 10 minutes. Serve over whole grains, if desired.

Nutritional Analysis

CALORIES: 312, CARBOHYDRATES: 64G, FIBER: 19G, TOTAL FAT: 2G, SATURATED FAT: 0G, PROTEIN: 14G

Note: Frozen vegetable mixes are a busy cook's shortcut. Stock up on bags of onion/green pepper/red pepper strips; you can use them any time you don't want to chop onions and peppers.

Dr. Gabe's Famous
Bean-Eggplant-Tomato Casserole . . . .

6 SERVINGS

1 onion, chopped
2 garlic cloves, minced
1 green bell pepper, chopped
1 (28-ounce) can Italian plum tomatoes, undrained and
*   chopped*
2 bouillon cubes
1 tablespoon dried oregano
Pinch of cayenne, or to taste
1 eggplant, cut into ½-inch cubes
2 (16-ounce) cans kidney beans, undrained
Cooked whole grains of your choice

Combine the onions, garlic, bell pepper, tomatoes, bouillon cubes, oregano, and cayenne in a large pot. Bring to a boil, reduce the heat, and simmer while dicing the eggplant. Add the eggplant to the pot and simmer 10 to 20 minutes. Stir in the beans and heat through. Serve over cooked whole grains.

Nutritional Analysis

CALORIES: 286, CARBOHYDRATES: 59G, FIBER: 18, TOTAL FAT: 2G, SATURATED FAT: 0G, PROTEIN: 14G

Note: Whole grains are interchangeable in most recipes. Use what you like best or whatever you have on hand.

Fastest Beans and Rice · · · · · · · · · · · · · · · · · · ·

4 SERVINGS

1 (16-ounce) can black beans, undrained
2 cups cooked brown rice or other whole grains
1 teaspoon mild chili powder
Pinch of cayenne, or to taste
2 teaspoons bouillon granules or 2 bouillon cubes, crushed
¼ cup chopped Italian parsley or cilantro leaves

Combine all the ingredients in a large pot, bring to a boil, and simmer 3 to 5 minutes. You can also cook the dish in a microwave oven for 3 minutes.

Nutritional Analysis

CALORIES: 199, CARBOHYDRATES: 38G, FIBER: 8G, TOTAL FAT: 2G, SATURATED FAT: 0G, PROTEIN: 9G

Paprika Casserole ·

6 SERVINGS

1 large onion, chopped
4 garlic cloves, minced
2 cups bouillon (see page 198)
2 carrots, sliced
2 medium red potatoes, cut into ½-inch chunks
2 tablespoons sweet paprika
2 bay leaves
Pinch of cayenne pepper, or to taste
½ cup dry sherry (optional)
1 red bell pepper, cut into ½-inch chunks
2 (8-ounce) containers mushrooms, quartered if large
1 (14-ounce) can artichokes, drained and cut into bite-size
  pieces
1 cup frozen peas
Cooked whole grains of your choice

Combine the onion, garlic, and bouillon in a large pot. Bring to a boil, reduce the heat, and simmer 5 minutes while preparing the other vegetables. Add the carrots, potatoes, paprika, bay leaves, cayenne, and sherry, if using. Return the liquid to boiling, then reduce the heat and simmer until the vegetables are just tender. Add the bell pepper, mushrooms, and artichokes and simmer 5 to 10 minutes. Stir in the peas and serve over whole grains.

Nutritional Analysis

CALORIES: 285, CARBOHYDRATES: 57G, FIBER: 13G, TOTAL FAT: 2G,
SATURATED FAT: 0G, PROTEIN 12G

Note: This recipe and many others can be cooked on the stove top, in a Crock-Pot or slow cooker, or in a covered casserole in a 375-degree oven. Stir occasionally and check to see if the potatoes are tender.

Penang Shrimp Curry . . . .

8 SERVINGS

8 cups water
2 pounds shrimp
2 onions, chopped
1 garlic clove, minced
2 celery stalks, chopped
1 carrot, chopped
1 tart apple, cored and chopped
1 green bell pepper, chopped
4 bouillon cubes
½ cup dry rolled or quick-cooking oats
1 tablespoon curry powder
½ teaspoon nutmeg
Pinch of cayenne pepper, or to taste
½ cup chopped basil, mint, or Italian parsley leaves, or some of
    each
Juice and grated zest of 1 lime
2 cups soy milk, light coconut milk, or yogurt (see Note on
    page 234)
Cooked whole grains of your choice

Garnishes
Grated coconut
Spanish peanuts
Jarred mango chutney

Bring the water to a boil in a large pot. Add half the shrimp and cook until they just turn pink, about 3 minutes. Remove them with a slotted spoon and place them in a colander to drain. Return the liquid to boiling and cook the remaining shrimp the same way. While you chop the vegetables, let the water continue to boil until it is reduced to about 4 cups. Add the onion, garlic, celery, carrot, apple, bell pepper, bouillon cubes, oatmeal, curry powder, nutmeg, cayenne, and basil. Reduce the heat and simmer, uncovered, at least 30 minutes (more won't hurt).

Peel the shrimp. When ready to serve, stir in the shrimp, lime juice, and the soy milk or coconut milk. Ladle over cooked whole grains. Arrange the garnishes in small bowls so guests can add their own.

Nutritional Analysis

CALORIES: 250, CARBOHYDRATES: 24G, FIBER: 5G, TOTAL FAT: 5G, SATURATED FAT: 1G, PROTEIN: 28G

Quick Chickpea Curry . . . .

6 SERVINGS

1 (16-ounce) package frozen pepper-onion mixture
2 (16-ounce) cans chickpeas, undrained
2 cups Italian plum tomatoes and their juice,
    chopped
2 bouillon cubes
1 tablespoon curry powder
Pinch of cayenne, or to taste
1 (10-ounce) bag baby spinach leaves
Cooked barley or brown rice

Combine all the ingredients except the grains in a large pot, bring to a boil, and simmer, stirring occasionally and making sure the bouillon cubes are dissolved, 5 to 10 minutes. Serve over the whole grains.

Nutritional Analysis

CALORIES: 260, CARBOHYDRATES: 49G, FIBER: 13G, TOTAL FAT: 4G, SATURATED FAT: 0G, PROTEIN: 11G

Quick Vegetable Curry . . . .

6 SERVINGS

2 (16-ounce) bags frozen stir-fry vegetables
½ cup bouillon (see page 198)
1 tablespoon mild curry powder
Pinch of cayenne, or to taste
1 (16-ounce) can chickpeas, undrained
Juice of 1 lime
2 cups light coconut milk or yogurt
Cooked whole grains of your choice
Jarred mango chutney (optional)

Combine the frozen vegetables, bouillon, curry, and cayenne in a large pot. Bring to a boil, reduce the heat and simmer, covered, until the vegetables are crisp-tender, 5 to 10 minutes (check the package for suggested time). Stir in the chickpeas and the lime juice. Add the coconut milk. (If using yogurt, stir it in just before serving. Do not allow the mixture to boil after you add the yogurt.) Serve over whole grains, with chutney on the side, if desired.

Variation: Add shrimp or other seafood of your choice.

Nutritional Analysis

CALORIES: 260, CARBOHYDRATES: 54G, FIBER: 12G, TOTAL FAT: 2G,
SATURATED FAT: 0G, PROTEIN: 10G

Note: If you add yogurt to boiling liquid it will separate and curdle. This doesn't harm the flavor but if you want a smooth texture you can do one of two things: Stir one tablespoon of cornstarch into the yogurt before adding it, or turn down the heat and don't let the pot boil again after adding the yogurt.

Shrimp with Wild Rice

6 SERVINGS

4 cups water
1 bay leaf
1 tablespoon Cajun spice blend
1 pound shrimp
1 onion, chopped
1 green bell pepper, chopped
3 celery stalks, chopped
2 garlic cloves, minced
Pinch of cayenne or dash of hot pepper sauce, to taste
1 (28-ounce) can Italian plum tomatoes, undrained and
    chopped
4 cups cooked wild rice or brown rice blend
1 bunch green onions, chopped
¼ cup chopped Italian parsley leaves
Freshly ground black pepper, to taste
Lemon wedges for garnish
Bottled hot pepper sauce, to taste

Bring the water, bay leaf, and Cajun spice blend to a boil in a large pot, add half of the shrimp, and cook until they just turn pink, about 2 minutes. Remove them with a slotted spoon and place them in a colander to drain. Return the liquid to boiling and cook the remaining shrimp the same way. Strain the cooking liquid and return 1 cup of it to the pot. Bring the liquid to a boil, add the onion, bell pepper, celery, garlic, tomatoes, and cayenne and simmer until they are tender, 10 to 15 minutes. Meanwhile, peel the shrimp.

Stir in the cooked wild rice, green onions, and parsley and cook 5 minutes. Add the shrimp just before serving. Season with pepper. Serve the lemon wedges and hot pepper sauce on the side.

Nutritional Analysis

CALORIES: 240, CARBOHYDRATES: 36G, FIBER: 5G, TOTAL FAT: 2G, SATURATED FAT: 0G, PROTEIN: 23G

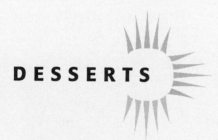

DESSERTS

Banana Rice Pudding

6 SERVINGS

2 to 4 ripe bananas, sliced

2 cups cooked brown rice, barley, or leftover cooked oatmeal

2 tablespoons brown sugar (diabetics can use an artificial sweetener)

¼ teaspoon vanilla extract
¼ teaspoon ground cinnamon

Combine all the ingredients in a microwavable dish and microwave on high for 3 to 4 minutes, or until the bananas are soft and the grains are heated through. Stir and serve.

Nutritional Analysis

CALORIES: 163, CARBOHYDRATES: 38G, FIBER: 3G, TOTAL FAT: 1G, SATURATED FAT: 0G, PROTEIN: 2G

Easy Banana-Strawberry Sherbet · · · · · · · · · · ·

4 SERVINGS

4 bananas
1 cup sliced strawberries, fresh or frozen, plus some for garnish
½ cup skim milk or soy milk

Peel the bananas, place them in a plastic bag, and freeze until firm. When ready to serve, slice the bananas into chunks. Place them along with the strawberries and the milk in a blender or food processor and puree until smooth. Spoon into dessert dishes and garnish with strawberries.

Nutritional Analysis

CALORIES: 131, CARBOHYDRATES: 33G, FIBER: 5G, TOTAL FAT: 0G, SATURATED FAT: 0G, PROTEIN: 2G

Note: Whenever you have bananas that are getting too ripe, peel them, put them in a plastic bag, and pop them in the freezer. That way you'll always have them on hand to make smoothies and quick fruit ices.

Fall Fruit Curry

6 SERVINGS

1 cup bouillon (see page 198)
1 teaspoon curry powder
1 teaspoon ground cinnamon
1 tablespoon grated fresh gingerroot
4 tart apples, cored and cut into bite-size pieces
2 pears, cored and cut into bite-size pieces
2 cups fresh or frozen peaches, cut into bite-size pieces
1 cup fresh or canned pineapple, cut into bite-size pieces
½ cup dried cherries or cranberries
Cooked barley or other whole grains (optional)

Combine all the ingredients except the optional grains in a large pot. Bring to a boil, reduce the heat, and simmer until the fruits are soft and their juices have thickened, 20 to 30 minutes. Serve over whole grains, if desired.

Nutritional Analysis
CALORIES: 262, CARBOHYDRATES: 59G, FIBER: 11G, TOTAL FAT: 2G, SATURATED FAT: 1G, PROTEIN: 6G

Gingered Fruit Compote . . . .

4 SERVINGS

> 4 slices candied ginger, cut into ¼-inch matchsticks
> 1 small pineapple, peeled, cored, and cut into bite-size pieces
> 2 bananas, peeled and sliced
> 2 large or 4 small tangerines, peeled and sectioned
> 1 cup raspberries
> 2 kiwifruit, peeled and sliced

Combine all the ingredients in a glass serving bowl. Chill until ready to serve.

Nutritional Analysis

CALORIES: 277, CARBOHYDRATES: 70G, FIBER: 8G, TOTAL FAT: 1G, SATURATED FAT: 0G, PROTEIN: 2G

Note: Candied ginger turns just about any combination of fruits into party fare. You'll find it in the Asian or gourmet section of the supermarket or in Asian groceries.

Fruit Kabobs . . . .

4 SERVINGS

> 2 slightly green bananas, cut into 1-inch pieces
> 1 cup fresh or canned pineapple chunks
> 4 star fruit, cut into ¼-inch slices
> 1 papaya, peeled and cut into 1-inch cubes
> 2 tablespoons lime juice (optional)
> 2 tablespoons lemon juice (optional)

Thread the chunks of fruit on 8 to 12 skewers. Serve raw. If you like, combine the lemon and lime juices and brush on the kabobs. Broil for 3 minutes, turn and baste, and broil 2 minutes more.

Nutritional Analysis

CALORIES: 147, CARBOHYDRATES: 37G, FIBER: 7G, TOTAL FAT: 1G, SATURATED FAT: 0G, PROTEIN: 2G

Fruity Pebbles

40 SERVINGS

3 cups mixed dried fruits
1 cup finely chopped pecans
Grated zest of 1 lemon
½ cup toasted wheat germ, plus more for rolling
½ teaspoon ground cinnamon
2 tablespoons chocolate-orange liqueur such as Sabra (optional)

Pour the dried fruits into a food processor and pulse until evenly chopped. (If they are very dry, soak them in water for several hours or steam them in a countertop steamer for 15 minutes. Drain.) Combine the chopped fruit with the pecans, lemon zest, wheat germ, cinnamon, and liqueur, if using. Shape into ½-inch balls and roll in the additional wheat germ.

Variation: Roll the Fruity Pebbles in finely ground pecans instead of the wheat germ.

Nutritional Analysis

CALORIES: 52, CARBOHYDRATES: 8G, FIBER: 1G, TOTAL FAT: 2G, SATURATED FAT: 0G, PROTEIN: 1G

Hawaiian Smoothie

2 SERVINGS

> 1 banana
> 1 cup skim milk or soy milk
> 2 cups bite-size fresh or frozen fruit—berries, melon, peaches,
> pineapple, oranges, or whatever else you have on hand

Place the banana and milk in a blender and process until smooth. Add the remaining fruit and puree. Serve in tall glasses or in bowls with spoons.

Nutritional Analysis

CALORIES: 157, CARBOHYDRATES: 34G, FIBER: 10G, TOTAL FAT: 1G, SATURATED FAT: 0G, PROTEIN: 6G

Note: This can be a breakfast treat, a dessert, or a snack any time of day.

Indian Rice Pudding

4 SERVINGS

> 2 cups cooked barley or brown rice
> 1 cup vanilla soy milk
> 1/2 cup golden raisins
> 1/2 cup dried cranberries or cherries
> 1/2 teaspoon ground cinnamon
> 1/2 cup chopped cashews

Combine the barley, soy milk, raisins, dried cranberries, and cinnamon in a microwavable dish and microwave on high 5 minutes. You can also cook the pudding on the stove top in a medium-size pot over low heat 5 to 10 minutes. Stir in the cashews just before serving. Serve warm or chilled.

Nutritional Analysis

CALORIES: 310, CARBOHYDRATES: 52G, FIBER: 10G, TOTAL FAT: 10,
SATURATED FAT: 2G, PROTEIN: 9G

Pineapple Fruit Boats . . . .
4 SERVINGS

Fruit-filled pineapples work with any combination of your favorite fruit. They're prettiest if you have brightly contrasting colors. For a special treat, marinate the fruit in liqueur.

2 small, fragrant fresh pineapples
1 cup raspberries
1 cup green grapes
1 cup blueberries
¼ cup fruit-flavored liqueur (optional)

Slice the pineapples in half lengthwise. Cut out the pineapple, leaving a ½-inch shell all around. Remove the core, dice the pineapple, and mix it with the raspberries, green grapes, and blueberries. Stir in the liqueur, if using, and spoon the fruit into the pineapple shells.

Nutritional Analysis

CALORIES: 215, CARBOHYDRATES: 50G, FIBER: 6G, TOTAL FAT: 2G,
SATURATED FAT: 0G, PROTEIN: 2G

Trail Mix Oatmeal Pudding . . . .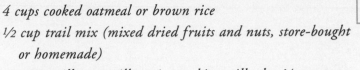
4 SERVINGS

4 cups cooked oatmeal or brown rice
½ cup trail mix (mixed dried fruits and nuts, store-bought
    or homemade)
1 cup vanilla soy milk or 1 cup skim milk plus ⅛ teaspoon
    vanilla extract

Combine the oatmeal and trail mix in a microwavable dish. Stir in enough of the soy milk to make a creamy consistency. Microwave on high for 2 to 3 minutes. Serve warm or at room temperature.

Nutritional Analysis:

CALORIES: 259, CARBOHYDRATES: 39G, FIBER: 5G, TOTAL FAT: 8G,
SATURATED FAT: 1G, PROTEIN: 10G

Tutti-Frutti Pudding . . . .
6 SERVINGS

1 cup vanilla soy milk or 1 cup skim milk plus
    1 teaspoon vanilla extract
½ teaspoon ground cinnamon
2 cups leftover cooked oatmeal or barley
¼ cup chopped dates
¼ cup chopped dried apricots
¼ cup dried cherries or cranberries
½ cup chopped pecans

Combine all the ingredients in a microwavable dish and microwave on high for 5 minutes. You can also add the ingredients to a small pot and heat gently on the stove top for about 10 minutes. Serve warm, at room temperature, or chilled.

Nutritional Analysis

CALORIES: 316, CARBOHYDRATES: 57G, FIBER: 11G, TOTAL FAT: 8G, SATURATED FAT: 1G, PROTEIN: 8G

SNACKS, APPETIZERS, AND SIDE DISHES

Almost-Instant Spanish Rice · · · · · · · · · · · · · · · · ·

4 SERVINGS

2 cups cooked brown rice or barley

1 cup tomato sauce

1 bunch green onions, chopped (white part only)

1 teaspoon chili powder

½ teaspoon ground cumin

½ teaspoon dried oregano

Pinch of cayenne pepper, or to taste

1 cup frozen peas

¼ cup sliced stuffed olives (optional)

Chopped cilantro or Italian parsley leaves for garnish (optional)

Combine the brown rice, tomato sauce, onions, chili powder, cumin, oregano, and cayenne pepper in a large pot. Bring to a boil, reduce the heat, and simmer 5 minutes. Stir in the peas and olives, if desired, and cook 2 to 3 minutes more. Garnish with cilantro or parsley, if desired.

Nutritional Analysis

CALORIES: 174, CARBOHYDRATES: 35G, FIBER: 6G, TOTAL FAT: 2G, SATURATED FAT: 0G, PROTEIN: 6G

Easy Spicy Peanut Dip

12 SERVINGS

> *1 cup crunchy-style peanut butter*
> *1 cup medium-hot jarred salsa*
> *¼ cup lemon juice, or to taste*
> *2 tablespoons Worcestershire sauce*
> *Bottled hot pepper sauce (optional)*

Combine all the ingredients in a bowl, using a fork to mash up any chunks of salsa.

Note: Serve with raw red bell pepper strips or any other vegetable dippers. You can make this as zippy or mild as you like, depending on the heat of your favorite salsa. Add a dash of hot pepper sauce if you want to turn up the heat.

Nutritional Analysis

CALORIES: 130, CARBOHYDRATES: 6G, FIBER: 2G, TOTAL FAT: 11G, SATURATED FAT: 2G, PROTEIN: 5G

Fresh Salsa

4 SERVINGS

2 ripe tomatoes, chopped
2 jalapeño chiles, seeded and chopped
1 red onion, chopped
1 garlic clove, minced
¼ cup chopped cilantro leaves
1 tablespoon lime or lemon juice
1 teaspoon ground cumin, or to taste

Combine all the ingredients and let the flavors blend for at least one hour before serving. This salsa keeps well if refrigerated in a covered container.

Nutritional Analysis

CALORIES: 33, CARBOHYDRATES: 7G, FIBER: IG, TOTAL FAT: IG, SATURATED FAT: OG, PROTEIN: IG

Hummus

6 SERVINGS

1 (16-ounce) can chickpeas, drained
1 small onion, chopped
1 garlic clove, minced
½ cup tomato sauce
Juice of 1 lemon
1 teaspoon ground cumin
½ teaspoon ground caraway seeds
Pinch of cayenne pepper, or to taste

2 tablespoons chopped cilantro leaves
Freshly ground black pepper, to taste

Place all the ingredients in a blender and puree until smooth. Serve as a dip for raw vegetables.

Nutritional Analysis

CALORIES: 110, CARBOHYDRATES: 22G, FIBER: 4G, TOTAL FAT: 1G,

SATURATED FAT: 0G, PROTEIN: 5G

Guacamole

8 SERVINGS

2 ripe avocados
2 tablespoons minced onion or 1 teaspoon minced garlic
1 jalapeño pepper, seeded and minced, or a dash of hot pepper
sauce (optional)
½ teaspoon salt
Juice of 1 lemon or lime

Cut the avocado in half and twist to separate. Discard the pit. Cut each half into thirds lengthwise. Remove the skin, place the avocado pieces in a bowl, and mash with a fork. Mix in the onions, pepper, if desired, salt, and juice. Serve immediately. (Avocado starts to blacken quickly, within half an hour or so.)

Nutritional Analysis

CALORIES: 170, CARBOHYDRATES: 8G, FIBER: 5G, TOTAL FAT: 15G,

SATURATED FAT: 2G, PROTEIN: 2G

Note: The best avocado for guacamole or salads is the dark-skinned, pebbly Hass variety. If you buy firm, unripe ones, let them sit out for a few days to ripen. Never buy avocados that are soft because they are likely to be bruised.

Harissa Sauce Spice Mixture (Hot!)

YIELD: ABOUT ¼ CUP

2 tablespoons cayenne pepper
1 tablespoon ground cumin
1 teaspoon ground caraway seeds
1 garlic clove
½ teaspoon salt
¼ cup fat-free Italian salad dressing

Mix the dry spices in a small refrigerator container. Peel the garlic clove and press it through a garlic press into the dry spices. Add the salad dressing and mix well. Store covered in the refrigerator; it keeps indefinitely. Harissa is very hot!

Note: A little harissa goes a long way. Stir in a tiny bit while you cook, or let each person mix a little into his own portion of any vegetable or bean dish. Be sure to caution anyone who is not familiar with Harissa. You'll find more of my favorite spice blends and dozens of other heart-healthy recipes at www.healthyheartmiracle.com.

Worksheets

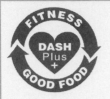

The Healthy Heart Miracle

BEFORE AND AFTER PROGRESS WORKSHEET

NOTE: *Shaded boxes indicate that following tests or measurements do not need to be taken.*

	My Target	Week 1	Week 3	Week 8	Follow-up (6 months or 1 year)
Weight _____					
BMI	Under 25 See page 10		■		
Waist/Hip	See page 11		■		
Inch of Pinch	Under 1" See page 12		■		
Blood Pressure	120/80 or lower See page 27				
Total Cholesterol	See page 24				
LDL	See page 24				
HDL	See page 24				
Triglycerides	150 or lower See page 26				
HBA1C	6.1 or lower See page 29		■	Recheck if abnormal	Recheck if abnormal
CRP	Negative See page 29		■	Recheck if abnormal	Recheck if abnormal
Homocysteine	40 or lower See page 31		■	Recheck if abnormal	Recheck if abnormal
Lp(a)	Negative See page 31		■	Recheck if abnormal	Recheck if abnormal

NOTE: *Lab values can vary. Your lab report will show the normal range for each test used by that lab. Check with your doctor for an explanation and restesting recommendations.*

To download this form, go to www.healthyheartmiracle.com.

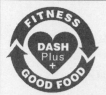

Choosing an Activity for Fitness

ACTIVITY_____ *(see page 33 for list)*

Make several copies of this worksheet and fill them out for each sport or activity you are considering. Tally your answers and you will see which ones fit you!

Skill Level
3 ☐ Easy, no skill needed.
3 ☐ Requires skill, but I already know how.

1 ☐ Need to learn new skill.
0 ☐ Too risky or too hard for me.

Convenience
3 ☐ I can do this at home.
2 ☐ I could do this nearby or in a convenient location.

1 ☐ I would need to travel to do this.
0 ☐ This would be too inconvenient for me to consider.

Equipment Needed
3 ☐ Need no equipment.

2 ☐ Need equipment, but it's inexpensive; I can buy it used or borrow it.

1 ☐ Expensive, but I think it could be worth fitting into my budget.
0 ☐ I could never afford this.

Enjoyment
3 ☐ I think this would be a lot of fun.
2 ☐ I might learn to like it.

1 ☐ This activity doesn't appeal to me.
0 ☐ I can't think of anything I'd rather do less.

Social Potential
3 ☐ I have a friend or group I could join to begin this right away.
2 ☐ I would enjoy finding and meeting other people who do this.

1 ☐ I would do this only by myself.
0 ☐ I would not enjoy the kind of people who do this.

Improvement Potential
3 ☐ I could start doing this now and grow with it. It's a good sport for novices and experts.
2 ☐ It's easy to start with some room to improve but not much of a challenge (e.g., exercise machine).

1 ☐ It's not a starter sport for me, but I could work on it and enjoy it later.
0 ☐ I don't fit into this picture.

Season/Weather
3 ☐ Year-round

2 ☐ I can't do this in bad weather, but I have an indoor backup plan (e.g., walking in a mall).

1 ☐ I could do this only a few weeks or months per year (e.g,, cross-country skiing).
0 ☐ This sport can't be done in my climate or location.

My Preference
3 ☐ Yes, this is definitely my choice.
2 ☐ Maybe I'll put this activity on my short list.

1 ☐ No. I might consider this later, but not for now.
0 ☐ No way. I would never do this.

My total score for this activity is _____

17–23 Close to perfect for me   **10–16 This has potential**
4–9 Maybe later   **0–3 Not for me**

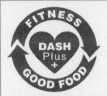

The Healthy Heart Miracle

DASH PLUS FITNESS LOG

Instructions

Use your Fitness Log to note each day's activities as you build your exercise program: what you did, length of time, distance, level of effort, how you felt, and any other helpful information.

You can use copies of this page or use any datebook or notebook. (See below)

If you are starting a new exercise program

❏ Get doctor's permission

❏ Complete Self-Assessment (page 15)

❏ Record physical activity every day

❏ Check local gyms, classes, etc.

❏ Complete exercise selection checklist (page 251)

Week _____

Sunday
Monday
Tuesday
Wednesday
Thursday
Friday
Saturday

To download this form, go to www.healthyheartmiracle.com

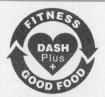

The Healthy Heart Miracle

DASH PLUS FOOD LOG

Instructions

Use your Food Log to note new recipes you tried that day, changes you made, foods you liked or didn't like, how you felt, shopping reminders, and any other helpful information.

You can use copies of this page or use any datebook or notebook.

Week _____

Sunday

Monday

Tuesday

Wednesday

Thursday

Friday

Saturday

References

BEFORE YOU BEGIN THIS BOOK

Hodson, L., et al. Maximal response to a plasma cholesterol-lowering diet is achieved within two weeks. *Nutrition Metabolism and Cardiovascular Diseases,* 2002, Vol. 12, Iss. 5, 291–295.

Jenkins, David J. A., et al. Effects of a dietary portfolio of cholesterol-lowering foods vs Lovastatin on serum lipids and C-reactive protein. *Journal of the American Medical Association,* 2003, Vol. 290, 502–510.

Roberts, C. K., et al. Effect of diet and exercise intervention on blood pressure, insulin, oxidative stress, and nitric oxide availability. *Circulation,* 2002, Vol. 106, Iss. 20, 2530–2532.

WEEK 1: WHAT'S YOUR RISK?

Bradley, Richard III, with Sarah Wernick. *Quick Fit, The Complete 15 Minute No-Sweat Workout.* Simon and Schuster, 2003.

Heim, D. L., C. A. Holcomb, and T. M. Loughin. Exercise mitigates the association of abdominal obesity with high-density lipoprotein cholesterol in premenopausal women: Results from the Third National Health and Nutrition Examination Survey. *Journal of the American Dietetic Association,* 2000, Vol. 100, Iss. 11, 1347–1353.

Hernandez-Ono, A., et al. Association of visceral fat with coronary risk factors in a population-based sample of postmenopausal women. *International Journal of Obesity,* 2002, Vol. 26, Iss. 1, 33–39.

Hu, F. B., et al. Prospective study of major dietary patterns and risk of coronary heart disease in men. *American Journal of Clinical Nutrition,* 2000, Vol. 72, Iss. 4, 912–921.

————. Television watching and other sedentary behaviors in relation to risk of obesity and type 2 diabetes mellitus in women. *Journal of the American Medical Association,* 2003, Vol. 289, 1785–1791.

Kahn, H. S., and D. F. Williamson. Abdominal obesity and mortality risk among men in nineteenth-century North America. *International Journal of Obesity,* 1994, Vol. 18, Iss. 10, 686–691.

Lawlor, D. Is housework good for health? Levels of physical activity and factors associated with activity in elderly women. Results from the British Women's Heart and Health Study. *Journal of Epidemiology and Community Health,* 2002, Vol. 56, 473–478.

Liu, S., et al. Fruit and vegetable intake and risk of cardiovascular disease: the Women's Health Study. *American Journal of Clinical Nutrition,* 2000, Vol. 72, Iss. 4, 922–928.

WEEK 2: WHAT DO YOUR TEST RESULTS MEAN?

Fung, T., et al. Whole-grain intake and the risk of type 2 diabetes: a prospective study in men. *American Journal of Clinical Nutrition,* 2002, Vol. 76, Iss. 3, 535–540.

Harding, A. H., et al. Fat consumption and HbA(1c) levels—The EPIC-Norfolk Study. *Diabetes Care,* 2001, Vol. 24, Iss. 11, 1911–1916.

Kannel, W. B. Historic perspectives on the relative contributions of diastolic and systolic blood pressure elevation to cardiovascular risk profile. *American Heart Journal,* 1999, Vol. 138, Iss. 3, Part 2, Suppl. S, S205–S210.

Kwiterovich, P. O. The metabolic pathways of high-density lipoprotein, low-density lipoprotein, and triglycerides: A current review. *American Journal of Cardiology,* 2000, Vol. 86, Iss. 12A, Sp. Iss. SI, 5L–10L.

Li, C. L., S. T. Tsai, and P. Chou. Comparison of metabolic risk profiles between subjects with fasting and 2-hour plasma glucose impairment: The Kinmen Study. *Journal of Clinical Epidemiology,* 2002, Vol. 55, Iss. 1, 19–24.

Siani, A., et al. The relationship of waist circumference to blood pressure: The Olivetti Heart Study. *American Journal of Hypertension,* 2002, Vol. 15, Iss. 9, 780–786.

Smith, G. D., et al. Leg length, insulin resistance, and coronary heart disease risk: The Caerphilly Study. *Journal of Epidemiology and Community Health,* 2001, Vol. 55, Iss. 12, 867–872.

Stavenow, L., and T. Kjellstrom. Influence of serum triglyceride levels on the risk for myocardial infarction in 12,510 middle aged males: interaction with serum cholesterol. *Atherosclerosis,* 1999, Vol. 147, Iss. 2, 243–247.

Superko, H. R. New aspects of risk factors for the development of atherosclerosis, including small low–density lipoprotein, homocysteine, and lipoprotein(a). *Current Opinion in Cardiology,* 1995, Vol. 10, Iss. 4, 347–354.

van Dam, R. M., et al. Dietary patterns and risk for type 2 diabetes mellitus in U.S. men. *Annals of Internal Medicine,* 2002, Vol. 136, Iss. 3, 201–209.

Verhoef, P., et al. Homocysteine metabolism and risk of myocardial infarction. Relation with vitamins B-6, B-12, and folate. *American Journal of Epidemiology,* 1996, Vol. 143, Iss. 9, 845–859.

WEEK 3: BLOOD SUGAR, INSULIN, AND REFINED CARBOHYDRATES

Camilleri, D. J., E. Chisholm, and W. Kraegen. Mechanisms of liver and muscle insulin resistance induced by chronic high-fat feeding. *Diabetes,* 1997, Vol. 46, Iss.11, 1768–1774.

Carmina-Lobo, E. The importance of diagnosing the polycystic ovary syndrome. *Annals of Internal Medicine,* 2000, Vol. 132, Iss. 12, 989–993.

Dandona, P., and A. Aljada. A rational approach to pathogenesis and treatment of type 2 diabetes mellitus, insulin resistance, inflammation, and atherosclerosis. *American Journal of Cardiology,* 2002, Vol. 90, Iss. 5A, Suppl. S, 27G–33G.

DeBerardis, G., et al. Erectile dysfunction and quality of life in type 2 diabetic patients—a serious problem too often overlooked. *Diabetes Care,* 2002, Vol. 25, Iss. 2, 284–291.

Han, D., et al. Insulin resistance of muscle glucose transport in rats fed a high-fat diet: A reevaluation. *Diabetes,* 1997, Vol. 46, Iss. 11, 1761–1767.

Kanauchi, M., N. Tsujimoto, and T. Hashimoto. Advanced glycation end products in non-diabetic patients with coronary artery disease. *Diabetes Care,* 2001, Vol. 24, Iss. 9, 1620–1623.

Knowler, W. C., et al. Reduction in the incidence of type 2 diabetes with lifestyle intervention or metformin. *New England Journal of Medicine,* 2002, Vol. 346, Iss. 6, 393–403.

Lazarus, R., D. Sparrow, and S. Weiss. Temporal relations between obesity and insulin: Longitudinal data from the normative aging study. *American Journal of Epidemiology,* Vol. 147, Iss. 2, 173–179.

Lebovitz, H. E. Rationale for and role of thiazolidinediones in type 2 diabetes mellitus. *American Journal of Cardiology,* 2002, Vol. 90, Iss. 5A, Suppl. S, 34G–41G.

McKeown, N., et al. Whole-grain intake is favorably associated with metabolic risk factors for type 2 diabetes and cardiovascular disease in the Framingham Offspring Study. *American Journal of Clinical Nutrition,* 2002, Vol. 76, Iss. 2, 390–398.

Norhammar, A., et al. Glucose metabolism in patients with acute myocardial infarction and no previous diagnosis of diabetes mellitus: a prospective study. *Lancet,* 2002, Vol. 359, 2140–44.

Pasquali, R., et al. Effect of long-term treatment with metformin added to hypocaloric diet on body composition, fat distribution, and androgen and insulin levels in abdominally obese women with and without the polycystic ovary syndrome. *Journal of Clinical Endocrinology and Metabolism,* 2000, Vol. 85, Iss. 8, 2767–2774.

Petersen, K. F., and G. I. Shulman. Pathogenesis of skeletal muscle insulin resistance in type 2 diabetes mellitus. *American Journal of Cardiology,* 2002, Vol. 90, Iss. 5A, Suppl. S, 11G–18G.

Pugh, J. Metformin monotherapy for type II diabetes. *Advances in Therapy,* 1997, Vol.14, Iss. 6, 338–347.

Reasner, C. A. Promising new approaches. *Diabetes Obesity & Metabolism,* 1999, Vol. 1, Suppl. 1, S41–S48.

Rett, K. The relation between insulin resistance and cardiovascular complications of the insulin resistance syndrome. *Diabetes Obesity & Metabolism,* 1999, Vol. 1, Suppl. 1, S8–S16.

Reusch, J. E. B. Current concepts in insulin resistance, type 2 diabetes mellitus, and the metabolic syndrome. *American Journal of Cardiology,* 2002, Vol. 90, Iss. 5A, Suppl. S, 19G–26G.

Schmitz, K. H., et al. Association of physical activity with insulin sensitivity in children. *International Journal of Obesity,* 2002, Vol. 26, Iss. 10, 1310–1316.

Truswell, A. S. Cereal grains and coronary heart disease. *European Journal of Clinical Nutrition,* 2002, Vol. 56, Iss. 1, 1–14.

Wursch, P., and F. X. Pisunyer. The role of viscous soluble fiber in the metabolic control of diabetes: A review with special emphasis on cereals rich in beta-glucan. *Diabetes Care,* 1997, Vol. 20, Iss.11, 1774–1780P.

Yki-Jarvinen, H. Combination therapy with insulin and oral agents: optimizing glycemic control in patients with type 2 diabetes mellitus. *Diabetes—Metabolism Research and Reviews,* 2002, Vol. 18, Suppl. 3, S77–S81.

REFERENCES

WEEK 4: BLOOD PRESSURE AND THE HIGH-PLANT (DASH) DIET

Appel, L. J., et al. A clinical trial of the effects of dietary patterns on blood pressure. *New England Journal of Medicine,* 1997, Vol. 336, 1117–1124.

Beevers, D. G. The epidemiology of salt and hypertension. *Clinical Autonomic Research,* 2002, Vol. 12, Iss. 5, 353–357.

Brzosko, S., et al. Effect of extra virgin olive oil on experimental thrombosis and primary hemostasis in rats. *Nutrition Metabolism and Cardiovascular Diseases,* 2002, Vol. 12, Iss. 6, 337–342.

Cole, C. R., et al. Heart-rate recovery immediately after exercise as a predictor of mortality. *New England Journal of Medicine,* 1999, Vol. 341, Iss. 18, 1351–1357.

Conlin, P. R. The effect of dietary patterns on blood pressure control in hypertensive patients: Results from the Dietary Approaches to Stop Hypertension (DASH) trial. *American Journal of Hypertension,* 2000, Vol. 13, Iss. 9, 949–955.

Edelman, D. A., and R. A. Paul. Does combination therapy with a calcium channel blocker and an ACE inhibitor have additive effects on blood pressure reduction? *International Journal of Clinical Practice,* 2000, Vol. 54, Iss. 2, 105–109.

Geleijnse, J. M., et al. Blood pressure response to fish oil supplementation: metaregression analysis of randomized trials. *Journal of Hypertension,* 2002, Vol. 20, Iss. 8, 1493–1499.

Hu, G., Q. Qiao, and J. Tuomilehto. Nonhypertensive cardiac effects of a high salt diet. *Current Hypertension Reports,* 2002, Vol. 4, Iss.1, 13–17.

Korhonen, M. H. Adherence to the salt restriction diet among people with mildly elevated blood pressure. *European Journal of Clinical Nutrition,* 1999, Vol. 53, Iss. 11, 880–885.

Leary, A. C., et al. The morning surge in blood pressure and heart rate is dependent on levels of physical activity after waking. *Journal of Hypertension,* 2002, Vol. 20, Iss. 5, 865–870.

McCarron, D. A., and M. E. Reusser. Are low intakes of calcium and potassium important causes of cardiovascular disease? *American Journal of Hypertension,* 2001, Vol. 14, Iss. 6, Part 2, Suppl. S, 206S–212S.

Miller, E. R. Results of the Diet, Exercise, and Weight loss Intervention Trial (DEW-IT). *Hypertension,* 2002, Vol. 40, Iss. 5, 612–618.

Moreno, J. A., et al. Effect of phenolic compounds of virgin olive oil on LDL oxidation resistance. *Medicina Clinica,* 2003, Vol. 120, Iss. 4, 128–131.

Ramachandran, S., et al. The lifetime risk for hypertension for middle-aged or elderly adults is estimated at 90 percent. *Journal of the American Medical Association,* 2002, Vol. 287, 1003–1010.

Resnick, L. M., et al. Factors affecting blood pressure responses to diet: The vanguard study. *American Journal of Hypertension,* 2000, Vol. 13, Iss. 9, 956–965.

Sacks, F. M., et al. Effects on blood pressure of reduced dietary sodium and the dietary approaches to stop hypertension (DASH) diet. *New England Journal of Medicine,* 2001, Vol. 344, Iss. 1, 3–10.

Swales, J. Population advice on salt restriction: The social issues. *American Journal of Hypertension,* 2000, Vol. 13, Iss. 1, Part 1, 2–7.

Tracy, R. E. Salt, obesity, and alcohol fail to induce a lasting rise of blood pressure with age, and may be independent of renocortical vasculopathy. *QJM, Monthly Journal of the Association of Physicians,* 1999, Vol. 92, Iss. 10, 601–607.

WEEK 5: ATHEROSCLEROSIS, FATS, AND FIBER

Albert, C. M., et al. Nut consumption and decreased risk of sudden cardiac death in the Physicians' Health Study. *Archives of Internal Medicine,* 2002, Vol. 162, Iss. 12, 1382–1387.

Connor, W. E. Importance of n-3 fatty acids in health and disease. *American Journal of Clinical Nutrition,* 2000, Vol. 71, Iss. 1, Suppl S, 171S–175S.

Davy, B. M. High-fiber oat cereal compared with wheat cereal consumption favorably alters LDL-cholesterol subclass and particle numbers in middle-aged and older men. *American Journal of Clinical Nutrition,* 2002, Vol. 76, Iss. 2, 351–358.

Desouza, C. Treatment with folate or vitamins B6 and B 12 lowers plasma homocysteine levels effectively. Drugs affecting homocysteine metabolism—Impact on cardiovascular risk. *Drugs,* 2002, Vol. 62, Iss. 4, 605–616.

Franceschini, G. Epidemiologic evidence for high-density lipoprotein cholesterol as a risk factor for coronary artery disease. *American Journal of Cardiology,* 2001, Vol. 88, Iss. 12, Suppl. S, 9N–13N.

Hardman, A. E. Role of exercise and weight loss in maximizing LDL cholesterol reduction. *European Heart Journal Supplements,* 1999, Vol. 1, Iss. S, S123–S131.

Hilbert, J. E., G. A. Sforzo, and T. Swensen. The effects of massage on delayed onset muscle soreness. *British Journal of Sports Medicine,* 2003, Vol. 37, Iss. 1, 72–75.

Hu, F. B. Fish and long-chain omega-3 fatty acid intake and risk of coronary heart disease and total mortality in diabetic women. *Circulation,* 2003, Vol. 107, Iss. 14, 1852–1857.

REFERENCES

Kashyap, M. L., et al. Long-term safety and efficacy of a once-daily niacin/lovastatin formulation for patients with dyslipidemia. *American Journal of Cardiology,* 2002, Vol. 89, Iss. 6, 672–678.

Kim, J. R. Effect of exercise intensity and frequency on lipid levels in men with coronary heart disease: Training level comparison trial. *American Journal of Cardiology,* 2001, Vol. 87, Iss. 8, 942.

Li, D. Omega-3 fatty acids and non-communicable diseases. *Chinese Medical Journal,* 2003, Vol. 116, Iss. 3, 453–458.

Libby, P. Managing the risk of atherosclerosis: The role of high-density lipoprotein. *American Journal of Cardiology,* 2001, Vol. 88, Iss. 12, Suppl. S, 3N–8N.

Lichtenstein, A. H., et al. Lipoprotein response to diets high in soy or animal protein with and without isoflavones in moderately hypercholesterolemic subjects. *Arteriosclerosis, Thrombosis, and Vascular Biology,* 2002, Vol. 22, 1852–1858.

Robins, S. J. Targeting low high-density lipoprotein cholesterol for therapy: Lessons from the Veterans Affairs High-Density Lipoprotein Intervention Trial. *American Journal of Cardiology,* 2001, Vol. 88, Iss. 12, Suppl. S, 19N–23N.

Sacks, F. M. The relative role of low-density lipoprotein cholesterol and high-density lipoprotein cholesterol in coronary artery disease: Evidence from large-scale statin and fibrate trials. *American Journal of Cardiology,* 2001, Vol. 88, Iss. 12, Suppl. S, 14N–18N.

Simopoulos, A. P. Essential fatty acids in health and chronic disease. *American Journal of Clinical Nutrition,* 1999, Vol. 70, Iss. 3, Suppl. S, 560S–569S.

———. Omega-3 fatty acids in wild plants, nuts and seeds. *Asia Pacific Journal of Clinical Nutrition,* 2002, Vol. 11, Suppl. 6, S163–S173.

Sinzinger, H. Statin-induced myositis migrans. *Wiener Klinische Wochenschrift,* 2002, Vol. 114, Iss. 21–22, 943–944.

Wrangham, R. Cooking and Human Origin. *Current Anthropology,* 1999, Vol. 20, Iss. 5, 567–594.

WEEK 6: INFLAMMATION, INFECTIONS, AND HEART ATTACKS

Albert, C. M., et al. The pravastatin inflammation CRP evaluation (PRINCE): Rationale and design. *American Heart Journal,* 2001, Vol. 141, Iss. 6, 893–898.

———. Prospective study of C-reactive protein, homocysteine, and plasma lipid levels as predictors of sudden cardiac death. *Circulation,* 2002, Vol. 105, Iss. 22, 2595–2599.

Albert, C. M., R. J. Glynn, and P. M. Ridker. Alcohol consumption and plasma concentration of C-reactive protein. *Circulation,* 2003, Vol. 107, Iss. 3, 443–447.

Bloemenkamp, D. G. M., et al. Chlamydia pneumoniae, Helicobacter pylori and cytomegalovirus infections and the risk of peripheral arterial disease in young. *Atherosclerosis,* 2002, Vol. 163, Iss. 1, 149–156.

Dugan, J. P., R. R. Feuge, and D. S. Burgess. Review of evidence for a connection between Chlamydia pneumoniae and atherosclerotic disease. *Clinical Therapeutics,* 2002, Vol. 24, Iss. 5, 719–735.

Folland, J. P. Fatigue is not a necessary stimulus for strength gains during resistance training. *British Journal of Sports Medicine,* 2002, Vol. 36, Iss. 5, 370–373.

Hoff, J., A. Gran, and J. Helgerud. Maximal strength training improves aerobic endurance performance. *Scandinavian Journal of Medicine & Science in Sports,* 2002, Vol. 12, Iss. 5, 288–295.

Hung, H. C., et al. Oral health and peripheral arterial disease. *Circulation,* 2003, Vol. 107, Iss. 8, 1152–1157.

Jenkins, David J. A. High-protein diets in hyperlipidemia: effect of wheat gluten on serum lipids, uric acid, and renal function. *American Journal of Clinical Nutrition,* 2001, Vol. 74, Iss. 1, 57–63.

McHugh, M. P. Recent advances in the understanding of the repeated bout effect: the protective effect against muscle damage from a single bout of eccentric exercise. *Scandinavian Journal of Medicine & Science in Sports,* 2003, Vol. 13, Iss. 2, 88–97.

Stewart, K. J., et al. Fitness, fatness and activity as predictors of bone mineral density in older persons. *Journal of Internal Medicine,* 2002, Vol. 252, Iss. 5, 381–388.

Wiesli, P., et al. Roxithromycin treatment prevents progression of peripheral arterial occlusive disease in Chlamydia pneumoniae seropositive men—A randomized, double-blind, placebo-controlled trial. *Circulation,* 2002, Vol. 105, Iss. 22, 2646–2652.

Ziegler, S., et al. Muscle cell proteins are selectively released into the blood stream by marathon running. *Acta Medica Austriaca,* 2003, Vol. 30, Iss. 2, 55–58.

WEEK 7: PREVENTING CLOTS, STROKES, AND DEMENTIA

Anderson, J. L., et al. Effect of implementation of folic acid fortification of food on homocysteine concentrations in subjects with coronary artery disease. *American Journal of Cardiology,* 2002, Vol. 90, Iss. 5, 536–542.

Barberger-Gateau, P., et al. Fish, meat, and risk of dementia: cohort study. *British Medical Journal,* 2002, Vol. 325, 932–293.

Ceriello, A., et al. Red wine protects diabetic patients from meal-induced oxidative stress and thrombosis activation: a pleasant approach to the prevention of cardiovascular disease in diabetics. *European Journal of Clinical Investigation,* 2001, Vol. 31, Iss. 4, 322–328.

Chiechi, L. M., et al. The effects of a soy rich diet on serum lipids: the Menfis randomized trial. *Maturitas,* 2002, Vol. 41, Iss. 2, 97–104.

Christensen, B., et al. Abstention from filtered coffee reduces the concentrations of plasma homocysteine and serum cholesterol—a randomized controlled trial. *American Journal of Clinical Nutrition,* 2001, Vol. 74, Iss. 3, 302–307.

Cui, J. H., et al. Cardioprotection with grapes. *Journal of Cardiovascular Pharmacology,* 2002, Vol. 40, Iss. 5, 760–767.

Jentjens, R., and A.E. Jeukendrup. Determinants of post-exercise glycogen synthesis during short-term recovery. *Sports Medicine,* 2003, Vol. 33, Iss. 2, 117–144.

Keijzers, G. B., et al. Caffeine can decrease insulin sensitivity in humans. *Diabetes Care,* 2002, Vol. 25, Iss. 2, 364–369.

Knekt, P., R Jarvinen, et al. Dietary flavonoids and the risk of lung cancer and other malignant neoplasms. *American Journal of Epidemiology,* 1997, Vol. 146, Iss. 3, 223–230.

Muntwyler, J., et al. Vitamin supplement use in a low-risk population of U.S. male physicians and subsequent cardiovascular mortality. *Archives of Internal Medicine,* 2002, Vol. 162, Iss. 13, 1472–1476.

Pan, J., et al. Niacin treatment of the atherogenic lipid profile and Lp(A) in diabetes. *Diabetes Obesity & Metabolism,* 2002, Vol. 4, Iss. 4, 255–261.

Pieper, J. A. Understanding niacin formulations. *American Journal of Managed Care,* 2002, Vol. 8, Iss. 12, Suppl. S, S308–S314.

Plat, J., and R. P. Mensink. Effects of plant sterols and stanols on lipid metabolism and cardiovascular risk. *Nutrition Metabolism and Cardiovascular Diseases,* 2001, Vol. 11, Iss. 1, 31–40.

Quere, I., et al. Red blood cell methylfolate and plasma homocysteine as risk factors for venous thromboembolism: a matched case-control study. *Lancet,* 2002, Vol. 359, Iss. 9308, 747–752.

Russo, P., et al. Effects of de-alcoholated red wine and its phenolic fractions on platelet aggregation. *Nutrition Metabolism and Cardiovascular Diseases,* 2001, Vol. 11, Iss. 1, 25–29.

Schachter, A., et al. High blood levels of insulin caused by resistance to the effects of insulin in people with polycystic ovary syndrome raises blood levels of homocysteine, regardless of body weight. *Human Reproduction,* 2003, Vol. 18, Iss. 4, 721–727.

WEEK 8: YOUR PERSONAL DASH PLUS LIFESTYLE PLAN

Binder, E. F., et al. Effects of exercise training on frailty in community-dwelling older adults: Results of a randomized, controlled trial. *Journal of the American Geriatrics Society,* 2002, Vol. 50, Iss. 12, 1921–1928.

Dey, S. K., et al. Coronary artery disease risk factors & their association with physical activity in older athletes. *Journal of Cardiovascular Risk,* 2002, Vol. 9, Iss. 6, 383–392.

Evans, W. J. Effects of exercise on senescent muscle. *Clinical Orthopaedics and Related Research,* 2002, Vol. 403, Suppl. S, S211–S220.

Gutin, B., et al. Effects of exercise intensity on cardiovascular fitness, total body composition, and visceral adiposity of obese adolescents. *American Journal of Clinical Nutrition,* 2002, Vol. 75, Iss. 5, 818–826.

Miller, G. E., et al. Clinical depression and inflammatory risk markers for coronary heart disease. *American Journal of Cardiology,* 2002, Vol. 90, Iss. 12, 1279–1283.

Stessman, J., et al. Effect of exercise on ease in performing activities of daily living and instrumental activities of daily living from age 70 to 77: The Jerusalem longitudinal study. *Journal of the American Geriatrics Society,* 2002, Vol. 50, Iss. 12, 1934–1938.

Wang, W. B. E., et al. Postponed development of disability in elderly runners—A 13-year longitudinal study. *Archives of Internal Medicine,* 2002, Vol. 162, Iss. 20, 2285–2294.

Resources

USEFUL WEB SITES

Healthy Heart Miracle

www.healthyheartmiracle.com

Resources, support, and community Web site for Dr. Mirkin's *Healthy Heart Miracle*. Download free tools, recipes, worksheets, and latest-breaking healthy heart information.

Dr. Gabe Mirkin on Health, Fitness, and Nutrition

www.drmirkin.com

Read or listen to hundreds of reports to help you maintain a DASH Plus lifestyle and understand the latest medical research.

American Heart Association

www.americanheart.org

Education and information on fighting heart disease and stroke.

American Diabetes Association

www.diabetes.org

Comprehensive information on diabetes, diabetes prevention, and treatment.

Blood Pressure and Heart Rate Monitors

www.lifewiseonline.com

LifeWise™ offers blood pressure, heart rate, and body fat monitors to help you keep track of your progress.

Exersage

www.exersage.com

Has photos of the stretches in Week 5 and the weight-lifting routine in Week 6, plus more helpful tips from former Olympian and coach Pat Connolly.

Heart Center Online

www.heartcenteronline.com

Web site for cardiologists and their patients, which includes a free e-newsletter on preventing and treating heart disease.

Heart Check America

www.heartcheck.com

Heart Check America provides coronary scans for the early detection of heart disease using Electron Beam Tomography (EBT) scanners.

National Heart, Lung, and Blood Institute

www.nhlbi.nih.gov

Information on heart, lung, and blood disease, including the latest research on lowering blood pressure and cholesterol.

Nutrition News Focus

www.nutritionnewsfocus.com

A free e-newsletter to help you interpret news stories on nutrition by the chairman of Nutrition and Food Science at Wayne State University.

Quaker® Oatmeal

www.quakeroatmeal.com

Learn how eating oatmeal every day can help you live a healthier life, as Dr. Mirkin recommends in *Healthy Heart Miracle*.

Quick Fit

www.ricksquickfit.com

Innovative program by fitness expert Rick Bradley for people who think they don't have time to exercise.

Resperate

www.resperate.com

Information on a non-drug medical device for therapeutic breathing exercises that can help to lower blood pressure.

Whole Foods Market®

www.wholefoods.com

The world's largest health-oriented food retailer offers nutrition information and recipes.

Index

Author, professor, columnist, former marathon runner, a practicing physician for forty years, and a radio talk show host for twenty-five, DR. GABE MIRKIN is recognized as a pioneer of the fitness movement in North America.

"Heart attacks, strokes, diabetes, and dementia are lifestyle diseases that often can be prevented with lifestyle changes," says Dr. Mirkin, a graduate of Harvard University and Baylor University College of Medicine. Dr. Mirkin sees about forty patients each day at his office in Maryland, and stays in touch with the latest findings by scanning as many as one thousand medical journals each month. He is one of a very few doctors board-certified in four specialties: Sports Medicine, Allergy and Immunology, Pediatrics, and Pediatric Immunology.

Dr. Mirkin wrote the chapter on sports injuries for the *Merck Manual* (both lay and physicians' editions), the largest selling book worldwide with more than one million copies in print. He has been the fitness broadcaster for CBS Radio News since the 1970s. He has written eight popular books, including *The Sportsmedicine Book,* the bestselling book on the subject that has been translated into many languages.

A Boston native, Dr. Mirkin did his residency at Massachusetts General Hospital, and over the years he has served as a teaching fellow at Johns Hopkins Medical School, assistant professor at the University of Maryland, and associate clinical professor in Pediatrics at the Georgetown University School of Medicine.

Dr. Mirkin ran marathons for many years and is now a serious tandem bike rider with his wife, Diana, often doing 40 to 60 miles in an outing.

DIANA MIRKIN is the director of Dr. Gabe Mirkin's Healthy Cooking School and manager of www.drmirkin.com. She has taught thousands of people how to make healthy foods taste delicious. Coauthor with Dr. Mirkin of *The Good Food Book, The Whole Grains Cookbook, The 20/30 Fat & Fiber Diet Plan,* and *Fat Free, Flavor Full,* she has developed hundreds of recipes that follow Dr. Mirkin's guidelines for healthy eating, featuring whole grains, beans, vegetables, and fruit.

Diana is a graduate of Vassar College and has an MBA from Loyola College. When she's not inventing tasty new recipes, she's usually out riding the tandem bicycle, gardening, or exercising her dogs.